REACHI

EXCELLENCE

in Healthcare
Management

REACHING EXCELLENCE

in Healthcare
Management

JOHN R. GRIFFITH ◆ KENNETH R. WHITE

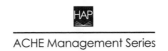

ACHE Management Series

Library of Congress Cataloging-in-Publication Data

Griffith, John R.
    Reaching excellence in healthcare management / John R. Griffith, Kenneth R. White.
    p. ; cm.
Includes bibliographical references and index.
ISBN 978-1-56793-364-2
1. Health services administration. I. White, Kenneth R. (Kenneth Ray), 1956- II. Title.
[DNLM: 1. Health Services Administration. 2. Quality Assurance, Health Care-
    methods. W 84.41]
RA971.G753 2011
362.1068—dc22
                                2010028735

The paper used in this publication meets the minimum requirements of American National Standard for Information Sciences—Permanence of Paper for Printed Library Materials, ANSI Z39.48-1984∞™

Acquisitions editor: Janet Davis; Project manager: Eduard Avis; Cover designer: Gloria Chantell; Layout: Putman Productions, LLC

Found an error or a typo? We want to know! Please e-mail it to hap1@ache.org, and put "Book Error" in the subject line.

For photocopying and copyright information, please contact Copyright Clearance Center at www.copyright.com or at (978) 750–8400.

Health Administration Press
A division of the Foundation of the American
    College of Healthcare Executives
One North Franklin Street, Suite 1700
Chicago, IL 60606–3529
(312) 424–2800

To the associates of the growing list of HCOs striving for excellence, with special thanks to those on the Baldrige journey.

Brief Contents

Detailed Contents

PREFACE

Reaching Excellence is a handbook for healthcare management professionals. It provides easily accessible summaries of best practices in all the areas of modern healthcare organizations—governance, clinical, logistic, and strategic operations. It is based on the actual practices of high performing HCOs and condensed from the award-winning text, The *Well-Managed Healthcare Organization*, 7th edition. It is a condensation for busy, knowledgeable managers who want the specifics without the detail.

Excellence means simultaneous high patient and associate satisfaction, strong earnings, and high quality of care. A growing number of American healthcare organizations (HCOs) have documented excellence. They all use the same management approach. They pay careful attention to a welcoming environment, continuous improvement of work processes, and a supportive culture. These make their organizations great places to work. Their loyal associates have the tools and the motivation to delight their customers and provide excellent care.

The common theme of these organizations, explained in Chapter 1, is that a specific culture (transformational and evidence-based management) and certain management activities (listening, measurement, benchmarking, negotiated goal-setting, and continuous improvement) are essential to high performance. To provide modern healthcare, specialized teams must complete specified tasks correctly to measured standards. Only some of these teams are directly involved in patient care. The balance provide clinical (e.g., laboratory, pharmacy, imaging), logistic (e.g., information, personnel, training, supplies) or strategic (e.g., planning, community relations, enterprise-level goals, finance, decision processes, culture) support that allows clinical teams to achieve excellence (see Exhibit 1.1). They are all essential; failure in one inevitably impairs the whole.

Reaching Excellence identifies and answers 160 questions on any HCO's path to excellence. It is organized similarly to actual large HCOs:

Leadership—the critical activities of the leadership team:

Chapter 1: integrating the HCO with its environment

Chapter 2: sustaining the organization culture

Chapter 3: maintaining the core operations that allow the teams to interact and coordinate effectively

Chapter 4: building and keeping an effective governing board

Clinical Operations—five chapters on core clinical functions:

Chapter 5: implementing 21st century care as a multi-team activity

Chapter 6: building and retaining a strong medical staff

Chapter 7: achieving Magnet-level nursing performance and nursing loyalty

Chapter 8: supporting excellent clinical support

Chapter 9: community health, going beyond excellent medical care

Logistic and Strategic Operations—six chapters on the "off stage" operations essential for excellence:

> Chapter 10: getting the right information to the right people at the right time
>
> Chapter 11: recruiting, training, rewarding, and retaining a high performance workforce
>
> Chapter 12: using the environment of care as a marketing weapon
>
> Chapter 13: expanding accounting and finance to provide cost analysis, goal-setting assistance, and fail-safe auditing
>
> Chapter 14: getting the most from an internal consulting resource and external consultants
>
> Chapter 15: integrating marketing and strategy to win market dominance

Each chapter addresses the "must do" questions fundamental to the success of the whole HCO. The structure of *Reaching Excellence* parallels its parent work, *The Well-Managed Healthcare Organization*, 7th edition. That work is a useful reference for amplification and documentation.

JRG
University of Michigan, Ann Arbor, Michigan

KRW
Virginia Commonwealth University, Richmond, Virginia

May, 2010

Chapter 1   In a Few Words . . .

Reaching Excellence is a handbook for healthcare management professionals. *Excellence* means simultaneous high patient satisfaction, high associate satisfaction, strong earnings, and high quality of care. A growing number of American healthcare organizations (HCOs) have documented excellence. They all use the same management approach. They pay careful attention to a welcoming environment, continuous improvement of work processes, and a supportive culture. These make their organizations great places to work. Their loyal associates have the tools and the motivation to delight their customers and provide excellent care.

High performing HCOs use objective measures extensively. They use rewards of all kinds generously. A "pretty good" HCO on the journey to excellence can see gains in year two, and substantial gains in year three.

Reaching Excellence is organized around the questions arising in real HCOs and is backed by the highly regarded text, *The Well-Managed Healthcare Organization,* 7th edition. The knowledge and skill in *Reaching Excellence* is the professional portfolio of healthcare management.

Introduction: What Is an Excellent Healthcare Organization?

Is This Your HCO?

You like your job, and the people you work with, but sometimes it's frustrating:

- It's hard to find the money for new equipment.
- Unpredictable absenteeism sometimes overworks the remaining staff.
- There's good quality overall, but a few patients don't get what they could.
- Patients like the hospital, but they don't always check the "top box."

That's the "pretty good" healthcare organization—doing well but could be better.

Reaching Excellence will tell you how to get better. This short chapter tells you what the model is, and how to start. Believe it or not, when you implement this model, you'll like your job even more.

What to Do Next?

Senior management and a few leaders on the board and medical staff buy the concept, "We're good, but we could be better." What should you do next?

Your coach says:

> What's needed is a snowball process that gets more and more people thinking about the concept. The recommended way to do it is called the "visioning exercise." Set up a special board/staff visioning committee. The board chair or the CEO might like to chair, but any senior leader can do it. The committee's charge is to review the organization's mission, vision, and values and revise them as necessary to expand understanding and consensus on what brings us together. It spins off subcommittees for various constituencies, so that panels from each constituency get to say what they'd like, and what they think current strengths and opportunities are. The committee pulls all this together—it's not as hard as it looks—and recommends a revised mission, vision, and values to the board. When the board accepts them, they are widely publicized and frequently referenced. They become real, not window dressing. The gain is not so much the wording as the learning. A whole lot of people grasp what the HCO's mission really is, and why.

Let's say you run a "pretty good" healthcare organization (HCO) and you want to make it better. *Reaching Excellence* can be your handbook. It summarizes what each "mission critical" activity must do if the whole is to succeed. It answers the "Frequently Recurring Questions" that arise as the activity strives for excellence in fulfilling its purpose. HCOs are not simple. There are a lot of activities that are essential to the whole. The core questions for the major activities, and the corresponding chapters, are listed on the next page.

All these activities must be performed effectively as a whole. Little failures can cause big problems in HCOs. Personnel shortages,

Chapter	Topic	Core Question
1	Beginnings	What is "excellence"?
2	Cultural Foundations	What are the climate and lifestyle of excellent HCOs?
3	Operational Foundations	What is the high performance "way we do things here"?
4	Governance	How does the board set realistic standards and goals?
5	Clinical Care	How do we approach patient care?
6	Medical Staff	How do we help every doctor be a great doctor?
7	Nursing	How can we be "a great place to give care"?
8	Clinical Support Services	What is excellence in labs, pharmacy, emergency department, etc.?
9	Community Health	Can our HCO build a healthier community?
10	Knowledge Management	What is the plan for information and learning?
11	Human Resources Management	How do we select, train, support, and develop our associates?
12	Environment of Care	How can we be sure our HCO is always safe, comfortable, and effective?
13	Finance	How do we earn surplus and invest it wisely?
14	Internal Consulting	How do we analyze opportunities and improve performance?
15	Marketing and Strategy	How do we make sure the HCO meets the real market needs?

misleading instructions, parking problems, communications break-downs, supply and equipment failures, and other problems create stress, and stress is the enemy of excellence.

WHAT IS EXCELLENCE?

Excellence for HCOs is high quality of care, high patient and associate satisfaction, and strong earnings. As shown in Exhibit 1.1, excellence is an ongoing process, a journey, not a destination. The journey builds a welcoming environment and sound work processes, giving well-trained associates a supportive environment that keeps them loyal and productive. It leads to a solid customer base and solid finances. The management challenge is how to sustain the loop, day in and day out. Excellent HCOs have solved that challenge.

In excellent HCOs the caregiving teams, doctors, nurses, and other associates delight their patients and are delighted themselves because the system works. Questions get answered. There are few or no personnel shortages. The equipment is up-to-date. The supplies are at hand. The building is comfortable. Team associates stay, and ongoing training makes them more effective. The teams improve quality, cut costs, and increase throughput. The result is excellent financial performance, and the gains are shared with the associates. In the words of one excellent HCO, St. Luke's of Kansas City, associates think it's the "best place to give care," and patients think it's "the best place to get care."[1]

Excellence is evidence-based. It's factual, not guesswork. When excellent HCOs say a customer is "delighted," they mean the customer checked the top box on the satisfaction survey. They measure all the elements—equipment age, supplies turnover, building safety and comfort, staff turnover, staff development, costs, throughput, quality, and more. For every measure, there's a current goal. For every goal, there's a team looking not just at the current goal but at the ultimate goal, the benchmark, the best.

Excellence is rewards-based. Smiles, hugs, high fives, celebrations, recognition, and cash are rewards for goal achievement.

---

[1]St. Luke's Health System, Kansas City, MO. [Online information; retrieved 6/15/09.] www.saintlukeshealthsystem.org/slhs/System/Saint_Lukes_Health_System/hp%5Bc%5D.htm.

Exhibit 1.1 Process of Excellence

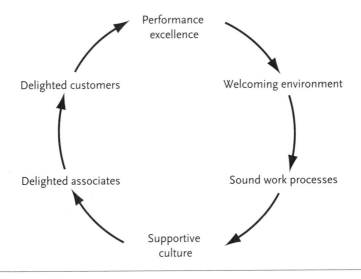

The goals are realistic. Progress is closely monitored, and management responds with help when problems are encountered. As a result, the goals are almost always met. Excellent HCOs are forward-looking—tomorrow's goals, not yesterday's problems.

CAN ALL HCOS BECOME EXCELLENT?

The count of documented excellent HCOs, places that can produce the numbers, is in the hundreds and growing. They include the recipients of the Malcolm Baldrige National Quality Award and other HCOs or systems that have been studied in depth. They cover a variety of settings, from Sharp HealthCare in San Diego to critical access hospitals in the Midwest. Collectively, they provide a broad spectrum of care, from traditional independent physician practice, through medical groups, ambulatory care centers, hospitals, rehab centers, home care, continuing care, and hospices. They exist in big cities and rural areas, with unions and without, with several different ethnic and religious cultures, with more than half the state Medicaid programs and regulatory bodies, and all major insurers. Of course they are all accredited by The Joint Commission, and all are Medicare participants.

There is no known roadblock to excellence. While the journey might be harder for safety net hospitals and clinics in challenging settings, there is no known reason why they can't make it, and no proven alternative path that's better.

WHAT IS THE PATH?

Any manager in an excellent HCO will say two things: "I work hard to make my team great," and "I love doing it." Over coffee, she might expand:

> This place is entirely different from what it was. It used to be okay. We were polite to one another, we did an okay job for our patients, but we didn't challenge each other. We didn't say, "Doctor, did you wash your hands?" We didn't take things apart and put them together better. We didn't celebrate our victories.
>
> We didn't have benchmarks. We didn't know that some places did things half again better than us. They had less personnel turnover. They had fewer infections, patient falls, needle sticks, lawsuits, and so forth. They had shorter stays. They had more 'delighted' patients, saying 'would return, would refer.' And they made more money.
>
> Of course, our HCO is now as good as any of the others. We're top decile in every one of those things. I can show you the graphs on our intranet.

The transition from "okay" to "excellent" takes a total rebuilding in most HCOs. Attitudes change, work habits change, procedures change. Change becomes a team sport and a way of life.

Excellent HCOs all do the same things. They build excellence on three major foundations as shown in Exhibit 1.2:

- Cultural: a commitment to values that attracts the respect and support of associates and patients
- Operational: a system that seeks out, evaluates, and implements opportunities to improve returns; and
- Strategic: a system that deliberately monitors the long-term relationships among stakeholders and responds to changing needs.

WHAT IS THE TIMETABLE?

The record suggests that a "pretty good" HCO can reach excellence in three years, on this timetable:

Year One: The focus is on the cultural foundations, building broad understanding about real commitment to values and the need to delight all stakeholders. Associate satisfaction measures begin to improve. Overall financial and operating performance does not change much, but previous performance is sustained. Scattered examples of quality, patient satisfaction, and efficiency appear.

Year Two: The focus is on improving basic operating systems, developing a planning and goal-setting mechanism, improving reliance on protocols and procedures, fixing major problems, and plucking the "low-hanging fruit." Performance measures begin to improve. In particular, quality should get better, stays shorter, throughput higher, and profit larger in at least a few service lines.

Year Three: The focus is on improving both the culture and the operating systems across the board. Stretch goals are set and achieved, bonuses paid, and most performance measures, including overall caregiver satisfaction, quality, and profit, are clearly improved.

Exhibit 1.2 Foundations of Excellence in Healthcare Organizations

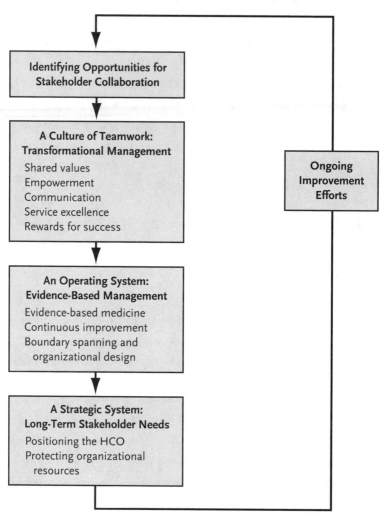

A few HCOs have moved to excellence within the three-year timetable from very challenging situations. They required drastic action: an unshakeable board commitment to progress, a senior management team united behind the effort, and unfortunately, the forced departure of a few highly visible people who did not understand or could not accept the foundations.

WHAT IS THE FOUNDATION FOR *REACHING EXCELLENCE?*

Reaching Excellence is a handbook for working HCO executives. It assumes a basic knowledge of what goes on and what the vocabulary is. It doesn't explain HIPAA or trace the history of physician privileges. It explains directly how excellent HCOs protect patient confidentiality—chapters 10 and 11—and build a strong medical staff—Chapter 6.

Reaching Excellence is based on *The Well-Managed Healthcare Organization*, 7th edition (also called *WMHO*, published in 2010 by Health Administration Press), a widely recognized textbook on HCO management. *WMHO* is designed for classroom use. It explains and documents extensively. The foundation for *WMHO* is the published and audited or peer-reviewed record of what excellent HCOs actually do. The chapters of *Reaching Excellence* deliberately parallel *WMHO*'s, making it easy to find support for a concept that's been challenged.

WHAT DOES EXCELLENCE MEAN FOR A PROFESSIONAL MANAGER?

The elements of management excellence are no mystery. They are specific, learnable knowledge and skills that successful professional HCO managers have mastered, and they are spelled out in *Reaching Excellence*. They are easy to begin. Mastery takes time and practice, but the payoff begins almost instantly.

The elements are a sound foundation for a 21st century professional career. The Board of Governors Examination in Healthcare Management, a requirement for acquiring the Fellow of the American College of Healthcare Executives (FACHE) credential, strives to evaluate them. The elements constitute the professional portfolio that managers bring to HCO conference tables. The doctor, the nurse, the lawyer, the accountant all arrive at those tables with portfolios of their own. *Reaching Excellence* and *WMHO* describe the manager's portfolio, practical knowledge of how to build sophisticated cultures and processes and how to make them attractive to associates and customers.

HOW CAN I USE *REACHING EXCELLENCE*?

Reaching Excellence provides a checklist on the details that support high performance. The chapters are kept as short as possible and are carefully action-oriented around questions that frequently arise among managers and teams seeking to improve HCO operations.

Here are some suggestions on how this book might be useful:

1. **We need to make clear why and how our culture is changing.** Some associate group—trustees, new first-line managers, union leaders, even the senior management team, or a couple of associates who seem not to understand—needs to be brought up to speed on what you're doing and why. Try Chapter 2. Its text is as clear as we can make it. Its exhibits are designed to support a brief meeting presentation. It describes a culture that is strikingly different from 20th century norms, from "Dilbert," and from too many HCOs. It describes a culture that's a major force to recruit and retain good people.

2. **Things aren't going well in _____ (fill in unit name).** Find the unit in the chapters. Each chapter outlines the functions essential to the *rest* of the HCO, including the unit's customers, and the measures that should be tracked and benchmarked. We've called that the *onstage* contribution. All HCO units have their own professional components and expertise, the *backstage* contribution. We've focused *onstage*, to identify information you can use a couple different ways:

    a. As a briefing to organize your questions before you meet the unit team.

b. As a summary you can share with the unit team to help its members explain to you where the opportunities for improvement (OFIs) are.

The latter path is often fruitful. The team knows the unit better than you ever will. The mandatory functions and the objective measures keep the conversation on a constructive path.

3. **We have a serious competitive threat.** Excellent HCOs expect to grow market share, not lose it. Competitors attack on two levels. They go after customers and your best associates. Go to the marketing and strategy chapter (15) for a background on maintaining market knowledge. Take a look across your satisfaction scores to identify your more exposed units, and go to those chapters. They'll need help improving their processes; we've summarized the support in Chapter 14. Because modern competition involves mergers and acquisitions, go to Chapter 4 to strengthen your governance.

4. **We have some opportunities for improvement (OFIs) in our clinical quality.** As Chapter 5 makes clear, clinical quality is an HCO-wide effort, involving medicine (Chapter 6), nursing (Chapter 7), clinical support services (Chapter 8), and logistic support services. The HCO is structured by service lines. Using these chapters, each service line can identify its own OFI profile and its OFI suggestions for other units. Collective bodies, like the senior management team, the Performance Improvement Council (Chapter 3), and the Medical Executive Committee need to integrate and prioritize the OFIs.

5. **We want to make the Baldrige journey.** That's great! Go for it! *Reaching Excellence* maps easily to the application. The Preface comes from your annual strategic assessment (Chapter 15); Leadership from Chapters 2 and 3; Strategy and Customers from Chapter 15 and Chapter 4. Knowledge Management and Human Resources Management have their own chapters in *Reaching Excellence.* Operations ties closely to Chapters 3 and 14. We can say without fear of correction, "All Baldrige recipients follow the approaches outlined in *Reaching Excellence.*"

Chapter 2   In a Few Words . . .

All reported excellent HCOs have carefully maintained a culture that deliberately delights both customer and provider stakeholders. Leadership under this culture has five functions:

- Promoting shared values by establishing, disseminating, and modeling attractive mission, vision, and values.
- Empowering associates so that they feel that they can change their work environment to improve mission achievement.
- Listening responsively to associates so that their needs are met and the responses model the organization's values.
- Supporting service excellence, helping delighted associates delight patients.
- Celebrating success and rewarding associates.

All leaders are trained to accomplish these functions and encouraged to work on their own advancement. Processes exist to stimulate the culture and deal with potential problems.

Building the Culture of Excellence

Is This Your HCO?

People are getting it! Empowerment means that everybody, not just the bosses, has the right *and the obligation* to fix things that reduce mission achievement. But there's some backsliding—it's hard to remember the new rules—and some disbelief, folks who don't think management really means it. What can you do about them?

The answer is "more of the same." Habits die hard. So you train, retrain, coach, and model. Especially model. Actions speak louder than words. Have a first-line supervisor who doesn't get it? Get her a coach at the same level. Send her to HR for more training. Have her superior spend direct time with her, helping her see the path. And for those who don't think you mean it, show them. Again, and again, and again.

What to Do Next?

Many of your managers will be happy with transformational management, and most others will catch on after they see it working around them. But "some dumb bunny never gets the word!" (A World War II expression, cleaned up a bit.) What should you do with the few who repeatedly fail to get it?

Your coach says:

> Treat this as a learning problem, and approach it with great, but not unlimited, tolerance. You train, re-train, coach, and model to help more and more people learn, reducing the slow learner pool. When it's clear that the culture is established generally and that the slow learners are a small and troublesome minority, make their position clear to them by loudly celebrating the record of those who are "in the know."
>
> At this point, you need to read Chapter 3. If their problem is not threatening operational performance (Exhibit 3.4) you can just let it go, but when it's holding their group back, or other groups back, you must act. Tell them directly: "Samantha, it seems like you're not fitting in the way you should. How do you feel about that? Would you be happier someplace else?" The second round is stronger; the third usually offers a termination plan. Note that under this strategy, when Samantha leaves, most people will be thanking you!
>
> Unfortunately, the "some dumb bunny" problem is pretty common. Many high performing HCOs have had to terminate a senior management team member. But only one. Samantha's departure helps a lot of people get on the bandwagon for good.

WHAT IS THE CULTURE ISSUE?

Culture establishes how an organization feels to customer and associate stakeholders. High-performing HCOs have built a new

21st century culture. It "empowers" all associates, and it is built around transformational (i.e., negotiation and persuasion) rather than transactional (i.e., authority and command) relationships. Every empowered associate is confident that she can change the work environment when it is necessary to achieve the mission. She expects answers, not orders, from her managers. Leadership must be responsive to associates; solutions must be negotiated, not imposed. The "service excellence" model shown in Exhibit 2.1 translates associate empowerment to better patient care and greater patient satisfaction when the culture is supported with a solid operating structure (Chapter 3).

The empowerment/transformational culture:

1. Makes HCOs attractive to doctors, nurses, and other associates. Associates want to come and want to stay. Personnel shortages are rare;

2. Creates greater commitment and enthusiasm among associates;

3. Translates that enthusiasm to customer service. The culture simultaneously improves patient and associate satisfaction and loyalty;

4. Makes change easier. The desirable changes are more readily identified and more readily implemented because associates "own" the change process; and

5. Is a radical change for many HCOs and many leaders. In terms of the comic strip, Dilbert is now empowered. He's working for the customer. The energies Dilbert and his colleagues once put into defeating the mindless bureaucracy now go to delighting the customer. The boss, the guy with the pointy hair, must answer Dilbert's questions and come to him for solutions. The excuses, evasions, secrets, power plays, and lies the boss previously used are no longer acceptable. Some former "bosses" find this transition pretty tough. Some don't make it.

Exhibit 2.1 The Service Excellence Chain in Healthcare

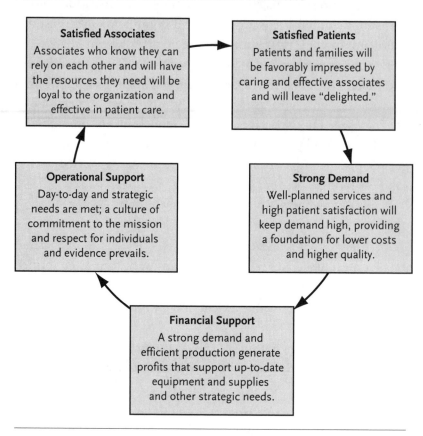

WHAT MAKES THE CULTURE EFFECTIVE?

Two forces make the transformational, empowerment, service-excellence culture effective. One is the energy and commitment released by empowerment. The other is the establishment of clear goals, not just overall, but in detail, so that every associate knows both the HCO's mission and his direct contribution to it. The culture is effective because the goals are clear and the tools to reach them are at hand. The culture—Chapter 2—goes hand in hand with operations—Chapter 3. Not only is management responsive, it's also effective. It gives honest answers to honest questions; it gives effective answers to achieve the mission. The "takeaways" are:

1. To reach excellence, your HCO must build a transformational, empowerment culture.
2. To maintain the transformational culture, all managers must learn to be responsive leaders. (Sometimes they are called "servant leaders.")
3. The transformational culture must be built simultaneously with an effective operating system.

HOW DOES AN HCO START ITS CULTURAL TRANSFORMATION?

The goal is the key. Empowerment releases energy; service excellence focuses the energy on the customer; the goal—what the customer wants and needs—is the organizing force. Cultural transformation begins with a "visioning exercise," a deliberate effort to get several hundred stakeholders to focus on the HCO's mission, vision, and values to understand them, to rewrite them if necessary, but most of all to remember them. A cascade of committees is used, starting with the governing board. The higher level committees debate and resolve disagreement. The final statement is by definition the consensus position, the "things on which we all agree." Once adopted, it's heavily promoted. It's on the wall, the website, badges, letterheads, newsletters, anywhere that people will see it and be reminded of it.

Several examples of missions, visions, and values are shown in Exhibit 2.2. Among excellent HCOs, there seem to be two prominent missions, "community service" and "excellent care." (We'll discuss the difference in Chapter 9. Community service includes excellent care.) The visions are the ideals for these concepts. The values conform to the Institute of Medicine's goals for 21st century healthcare: "safe, effective, patient-centered, timely, efficient, and equitable."[1] They also commit to more general virtues of respect and compassion. A commitment to "stewardship" is also common. They are consistent with widely accepted healthcare professional values of non-maleficence, beneficence, autonomy, and justice.

How does a "pretty good" HCO move to excellence?

1. It restates and re-commits to its mission, vision, and values. It uses the visioning process to build broad consensus on purposes.

2. The governing board adopts the concepts of the re-invigorated vision and accepts the challenge to move to excellence, recognizing that the changes will be profound, but setting milestones and anticipated completion dates.

3. The senior leaders agree unanimously to the effort. They begin the spread of the new culture by changing their behavior to reflect responsive leadership.

4. As the senior leaders "cruise and connect," they seek ways to demonstrate the power of a transformational culture and look for teams that can help as pilots and demonstration sites.

5. The success of pilots and demonstrations is widely celebrated and used to show the nature of the new culture and the HCO's commitment to it.

6. Coaching, modeling, and training are used deliberately to help other managers make the transition to responsive leadership.

7. Operational foundations and strategic protections are developed to support continuous improvement and evidence-based management.

The success of this strategy depends on two conditions. The first is consistent commitment. Many HCOs are afflicted with the "flavor of the month" approach to improvement. This year it's Lean; next year, servant leadership; everyone knows that the year after will be something different. Transformational management is

---

[1]Institute of Medicine Committee on Quality Health Care in America. 2001. *Crossing the Quality Chasm: A New Health System for the 21st Century.* Washington, DC: National Academies Press, p. 39.

Exhibit 2.2 Mission, Vision, and Values of Baldrige Award Recipients, 2002–2008

Organization	Mission	Vision	Values
SSM Health Care	Through our exceptional health care services, we reveal the healing presence of God.	. . . communities, especially those that are. . . marginalized, will experience improved health in mind, body, spirit and environment.	Compassion Respect Excellence Stewardship Community
Baptist Memorial	To provide superior service based on Christian values to improve the quality of life for people and communities served	To become the best health system in America	Integrity Vision Innovation Superior service Stewardship Teamwork
Saint Luke's	. . . highest levels of excellence in . . . health services to all patients in a caring environment	. . . best place to get care, best place to give care	Quality excellence Customer focus Resource management Teamwork

Continued

Exhibit 2.2 Continued

Organization	Mission	Vision	Values
RW Johnson	Excellence through service. We exist to promote, preserve and restore the health of our community.	To passionately pursue the health and well-being of our patients, employees and the community	Quality Understanding Excellence Service Teamwork
Bronson	Provide excellent healthcare services.	. . . a national leader in healthcare quality	Care and respect Teamwork Stewardship Commitment to community Pursuit of excellence
North Mississippi	To continuously improve the health of the people of our region	To be the provider of the best patient-centered care and health services in America . . .	Compassion Accountability Respect Excellence Smile

Exhibit 2.2 Continued

Organization	Mission	Vision	Values
Mercy	The Mission of Mercy Health System is to provide exceptional healthcare services resulting in healing in the broadest sense.	Quality—Excellence in patient care Service—Exceptional patient and customer service Partnering—Best place to work Cost—Long-term financial success	Healing in its broadest sense Patients come first Treat each other like family Strive for excellence
Sharp	To improve the health of those we serve with a commitment to excellence in all that we do Sharp's goal is to offer quality care and services that set community standards, exceed patients' expectations, and are provided in a caring, convenient, cost-effective, and accessible manner.	Sharp will redefine the health care experience through a culture of caring, quality, service, innovation, and excellence. Sharp will be recognized by employees, physicians, patients, volunteers, and the community as: the best place to work, the best place to practice medicine, and the best place to receive care.	Integrity Caring Innovation Excellence
Poudre Valley	To be an independent, non-profit organization and to provide innovative, comprehensive care of the highest quality, always exceeding customer expectations	To provide world-class health care	Quality Compassion Confidentiality Dignity/respect Equality Integrity

not an annual, it's a perennial. It takes time to grow, but its rewards are continuous. The board's and senior management's commitment at steps two and three must be for at least three years of diligent effort. Other programs can be added—the operational foundations provide several opportunities—but the transformational commitment must not be abandoned.

The second condition is the simultaneous move to strengthen the operational foundation and evidence-based management. Leadership and transformational culture are necessary, but not sufficient. Results require solid work processes. Even if I think my boss is great and the team is the best I've ever worked with, it's tough to improve if the staff is poorly trained, supplies are missing, and the record's unreliable. Those are results issues that the operational foundation addresses.

Step 4 calls for finding a willing pilot, a team that's an enthusiastic supporter of the mission. In that unit, the following take place:

1. The unit leadership is trained to responsive management and an empowerment culture.
2. Unit-level measures are established reflecting the unit's contribution to the mission, vision, and values.
3. The measures are implemented, benchmarks are found, and goals are set.
4. The unit identifies and prioritizes its opportunities for improvement (OFIs), using the benchmarks as guides.
5. Process improvement teams (PITs) identify new work processes that support better outcomes.
6. The new processes are implemented and the goals are achieved.
7. The unit looks for more OFIs, sets new goals, and continues the process improvement.

Each step is celebrated. Cash rewards—substantial bonuses in some cases—are appropriate at step 7. The celebrations are deliberately loud enough to attract attention from other units.

HOW DOES AN HCO EXPAND ITS TRANSFORMATIONAL CULTURE?

The model of transformational culture and service excellence is extensively documented. It works. In an HCO, the lesson that it works must be learned by several thousand people. The transition to the transformational culture is disruptive to the conventional order, and as a result, it can generate a substantial backlash. People who are used to having their word accepted without question sometimes have trouble listening and responding. People who have become comfortable working in authoritarian environments have trouble framing the questions they want to ask. To help people learn the lesson, several approaches are useful:

1. Find leaders who are doing it. Recognize them, and celebrate their contribution. Ask them to explain to colleagues.
2. Emphasize advantages that respond to specific needs. Service excellence supports patient satisfaction. It delights patients. Doctors' patients will be more pleased, as well as better cared for. Service excellence can be used to expand markets, including doctors' practices. It reduces nurse staffing problems (Chapter 7). It reduces clinical errors. It makes jobs more rewarding. Associates feel better at the end of the day. It is a foundation for reduced malpractice awards (Chapter 6). It allows people to earn bonuses.
3. Select expansion sites with care, and train leaders for their new roles. Keep coaching and modeling the desired behavior. Use the growing cadre of believers as a sales force.
4. Stay "on message" and keep repeating it. The transformational culture is a created environment that must be continuously sustained. The activities shown in Exhibit 2.4 are not "do once"; they are "do constantly." Step 6 leads to Step 1. Every OFI is potentially related to misunderstandings or failure in the culture.

5. Keep celebrations and rewards flowing. An honest answer is also a reward, particularly if it's well phrased. A celebration can be as simple as a high five. Successful HCOs celebrate every victory, and they have a lot of ways to reward. Bonuses are a reward; they are earned and affordable in high performance HCOs.

HOW DOES AN HCO MEASURE ITS CULTURE?

Every part of high-performing HCOs is measured and, wherever possible, benchmarked. Improvement goals are set, achieved, and rewarded. That applies to the culture and the leadership. Although measuring culture is challenging, culture is effective if:

- associate retention and satisfaction are high;
- recruitment shortages, accidents, and absenteeism are low;
- operating goals are met and moving toward benchmark;
- patients are satisfied; and
- market share is growing.

All of these dimensions can be measured, as shown in Exhibit 2.3. The measures support the continuous improvement of the culture. They indicate OFIs in individual units or larger aggregates.

Surveys of associate and patient satisfaction provide important information on the culture. In addition, each leader has an annual 360-degree or multi-rater review—a subjective evaluation by her superior, peers, and subordinates—to supplement the measures of unit performance. The combined information is reviewed with a superior to create a professional development plan using a mix of mentoring, special assignments, and continuing education. Leaders are held accountable for their professional development plans and for assisting less-experienced leaders in advancing their careers. Many organizations put a premium on

Exhibit 2.3 Measuring HCO Culture

Input Oriented	Output Oriented
Demand	*Output/Productivity*
Associate retention	Counts of training program
Personnel shortages	attendance and completion
Delays in filling positions	
Cost/Resources	*Quality*
Direct cost of training is	Quality of training programs is
measured and reported through	assessed by survey,
Human Resources.	examination, observation, and
Total cost of the culture is	later job performance.
difficult to estimate, because	360-degree reviews directly
many activities are integrated	measure leader capability.
with other work.	Achievement of unit goals
Human Resources	*Customer Satisfaction*
Associate satisfaction	Patient satisfaction
360-degree leader evaluations	Market share or demand
Leader satisfaction	
Leader retention	

diversity, advancing underrepresented groups, including women, to higher management levels, with a goal of incorporating the demographic characteristics of the community into leadership teams at all organizational levels.

Exhibit 2.4 shows how the leadership measures are used in a service excellence context. Careful judgment is important. For example, an operating unit is below benchmark on quality, productivity, or patient satisfaction, creating a mission-related OFI. A root cause question is, "Can the OFI be achieved by improving the culture?" The answer is suggested by the measures of associate satisfaction, retention, absenteeism, and safety. If none of these is below the comparable units, something else is probably the root

Exhibit 2.4 Relating Leadership and Culture to Mission Achievement

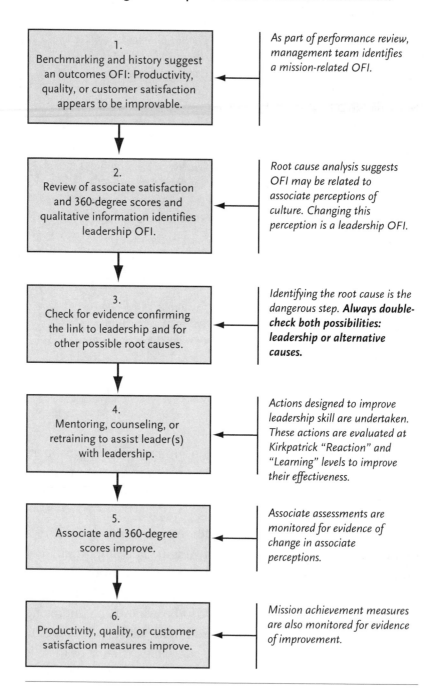

1.
Benchmarking and history suggest an outcomes OFI: Productivity, quality, or customer satisfaction appears to be improvable.

As part of performance review, management team identifies a mission-related OFI.

2.
Review of associate satisfaction and 360-degree scores and qualitative information identifies leadership OFI.

Root cause analysis suggests OFI may be related to associate perceptions of culture. Changing this perception is a leadership OFI.

3.
Check for evidence confirming the link to leadership and for other possible root causes.

*Identifying the root cause is the dangerous step. **Always double-check both possibilities: leadership or alternative causes.***

4.
Mentoring, counseling, or retraining to assist leader(s) with leadership.

Actions designed to improve leadership skill are undertaken. These actions are evaluated at Kirkpatrick "Reaction" and "Learning" levels to improve their effectiveness.

5.
Associate and 360-degree scores improve.

Associate assessments are monitored for evidence of change in associate perceptions.

6.
Productivity, quality, or customer satisfaction measures improve.

Mission achievement measures are also monitored for evidence of improvement.

cause. The professional response is to ask two further questions at step 3: How good is the evidence supporting the assumption that leadership is improvable? and What other possible causes might be contributing to the OFI?

WHAT DOES RESPONSIVE LEADERSHIP REALLY MEAN?

Power in traditional HCOs came from rank or professional stature. In the transformational management model:

Power and authority come from knowledge.

This is a major shift, because the people doing the work often have low rank or stature but profound insights into the work. That's why their questions must be heard and answered. That's how debate will be resolved: facts win. That's why the empowered organization does not degenerate into anarchy; everyone is committed to a common mission and bound by a common set of facts.

When a manager reverts to the old Dilbert games, the message to associates is "They didn't really mean it when they shifted to transformational leadership." Sharp HealthCare emphasizes its transformational commitment with positive reinforcement. It holds that to implement the mission, vision, and values, certain behaviors are essential. It expects these of all associates, but it expects all its managers, from first line to CEO, to model the behaviors. Here's the list:

12 Employee Behavior Standards

1. It's a Private Matter: Maintain Confidentiality
2. To "E" or Not to "E": Use E-mail Manners
3. Vive La Différence!: Celebrate Diversity

4. Get Smart: Increase Skills and Competence
5. Attitude is Everything: Create a Lasting Impression
6. Thank Somebody: Reward and Recognition
7. Make Words Work: Talk, Listen, and Learn
8. All For One, One For All: Teamwork
9. Make It Better: Service Recovery
10. Think Safe, Be Safe: Safety At Work
11. Look Sharp, Be Sharp: Appearance Speaks
12. Keep In Touch: Ease Waiting Times

5 "Must Haves"

1. Greet people with a smile and "hello," using their name.
2. Take people where they are going.
3. Use key words at key times: "Is there anything else I can do for you? I have the time."
4. Foster an attitude of gratitude.
5. Round with reason.

and, for all associates working with patients, an AIDET acronym:

A **Acknowledge:** Acknowledge people with a smile and use their names.

I **Introduce:** Introduce yourself to others politely.

D **Duration:** Keep in touch to ease waiting times.

E **Explanation:** Explain how procedures work and who to contact if they need assistance.

T **Thank You:** Thank people for using Sharp HealthCare.[2]

---

[2]Sharp HealthCare Malcolm Baldrige National Quality Award Application. 2007. [Online information; retrieved 12/16/08.]. www.baldrige.nist.gov/Contacts_Profiles.htm, Preface, pp. i–ii.

WHAT ARE SOME GOOD RESPONSES TO COMMON ISSUES?

Rounding and deliberately encouraging associate questions—"cruising and connecting"—require constructive responses. A lot of early questions fall into categories. The response paths and the subtexts involved are shown in Exhibit 2.5.

The transformational culture emphasizes negotiations. Negotiating not only resolves many concerns and disputes but also reassures associates that independent thought is a desirable behavior. If it leads to dispute, there will be a reasonable path to resolution. Some disputes will require additional attention by senior management and governing board members. What might be called "the appeals process" is driven by some agreed-upon principles:

1. *Evidence drives the decisions.* Objective measurement trumps tradition, status, and opinion. What is best for the patient is what is scientifically determined to be best. What is realistic for the associate is the best the associate can expect elsewhere.

2. *Negotiation is improved by patience, listening, and imagination.* Many apparent conflicts are actually misunderstandings. Careful listening expands understanding and reveals consensus opportunities. Imagination—thinking outside the box—identifies new opportunities to resolve apparently conflicting needs.

3. *Equity, not equality, drives the organization's ultimate position.* Under an equity concept, each stakeholder is treated fairly in terms of his or her contribution. Under an equality concept, each is treated equally. While the definition of contribution is never easy, the concept forces participants to recognize realistic differences in influence.

Exhibit 2.5 Frequently Negotiated Issues and Solution Paths for Excellent HCOs

Issue	Negotiation Path	Implications
"Unsafe situation"	"Thank you for noticing it. Security will evaluate it and will give you a report. When you get the report let me know if you're satisfied."	Value: Safety is critical for all associates. We don't tolerate unsafe situations. Fact: We use a trained team to evaluate risks, and we follow through.
"Need new equipment"	"We spend millions each year on new equipment, so we have a process of careful, competitive review. Units that show how the investment will improve quality, efficiency, or customer satisfaction usually get their requests."	Value: New equipment is important to fulfilling our mission, but money does not grow on trees. Fact: New equipment is justified based on specific improvements in important operational measures.
"Not enough nurses (or other staff)"	"That's a good question. We have a nurse staffing system, and we monitor benchmarks—what other excellent HCOs do—and patient outcomes. If you think your floor staffing should be changed, and your coworkers agree, we'll form a PIT to re-evaluate it."	Value: Enough nursing to assure quality and patient satisfaction is part of our mission, but so is control of costs. Fact: Staffing is set by a specific process that includes measures of effectiveness. The staffing process, like all others, is subject to continuous improvement.
"Disagree with the protocol"	"We use caregiver panels to select our protocols, and we try to follow the evidence-based medicine rules. The chair of your panel would like to know your concerns. I'll arrange a meeting."	Value: Science drives our clinical practice, but your opinion is important. Fact: Any protocol is a candidate for improvement. Suggestions are welcome and are evaluated in a careful process.

Exhibit 2.5 Continued

Issue	Negotiation Path	Implications
"This patient does not fit the protocol"	"Caregivers are expected to use their professional judgment to leave the protocol when indicated. We do ask for a note in the chart, so that others know what is being done."	*Value:* Care is patient-centered. Professionals are expected to exercise judgment. *Fact:* Judgment must be documented, both for effective communication and later review.
"My supervisor isn't fair"	"I'm sorry to hear that. Tell me more about your concerns, and we'll see how we can improve things."	*Value:* Associates are important stakeholders, but there are two sides to every argument. *Fact:* The HCO has a variety of training and counseling programs to resolve common sources of dissatisfaction, but using them requires a candid and thorough understanding of the cause.
"I want more money"	"Let's talk about that. We set our compensation carefully, and Human Resources can show you how we arrived at yours. We also offer bonuses, and you get a regular report on yours. One way to get more money is to win a promotion. Let's go over some steps you might take to do that."	*Value:* Compensation needs to be fair to all stakeholders. Associates are encouraged to improve. *Fact:* Compensation is based on an objective process. The HCO measures employee contribution, rewards effort, and encourages growth.

4. *Stakeholders and associates are free to terminate their relationship with the organization; conversely, the group as a whole can terminate its relationship with any stakeholder.* The usual goal is to retain and strengthen relationships, but it is occasionally necessary for some to seek separate paths.
5. *The governing board's calendar ultimately forces a decision.* The calendar is set for the good of the whole and is itself negotiated. Once set, it is a shared commitment that cannot easily be avoided.

Perhaps the most important of these is number five. It states that no single stakeholder or stakeholder group can hold the majority hostage. Even disassociation, reconfiguration, or closure is at some point superior to continued dispute, and it is the obligation of the governance structure, described in Chapter 4, to identify when that it so. Disputes rarely reach this level, but it is important to the long-run success of the transformational culture that such an outcome is a realistic, if remote, possibility.

CAN I DO IT? CAN I PERSONALLY BE A RESPONSIVE LEADER?

Transformational leadership is learned behavior. What this means for beginners in healthcare management can be summarized in four sentences.

1. The commitment, the will to succeed, is the important part.
2. Practice is the foundation for mastering competencies.
3. Guided practice, with appropriate training, coaching, and feedback, helps more leaders succeed, and succeed faster.
4. Regular review of competencies, identification of personal OFIs, and planned actions to improve are critical elements.

SUGGESTED READINGS

Collins, J. C. 2001. *Good to Great: Why Some Companies Make the Leap—and Others Don't.* New York: HarperBusiness.

Dye, C. F., and A. N. Garman. 2006. *Exceptional Leadership: 16 Critical Competencies for Healthcare Executives.* Chicago: Health Administration Press.

Kouzes, J. M., and B. Z. Posner. 2007. *The Leadership Challenge,* 4th edition. San Francisco: Jossey-Bass.

Lee, B. D., and J. W. Herring. 2008. *Growing Leaders in Healthcare: Lessons from the Corporate World.* Chicago: Health Administration Press.

Pfeffer, J., and R. I. Sutton. 2006. *Hard Facts, Dangerous Half-Truths, and Total Nonsense: Profiting from Evidence-Based Management.* Boston: Harvard Business School Press.

Chapter 3   In a Few Words . . .

Excellence requires a dynamic operational infrastructure that must be developed in parallel with the transformational culture. The infrastructure provides the rules and mechanics for continuous improvement. It:

- Drives systematic continuous improvement.
- Sets quantitative goals for all units.
- Provides the knowledge base for mission achievement.
- Identifies changes in stakeholder needs.
- Improves itself.

The infrastructure requires a strong system of logistic and strategic support services to meet the needs of operating units. Infrastructure effectiveness is as essential to excellence as an empowerment culture.

Building the Excellent Infrastructure

Is This Your HCO?

Your HCO does the functions in Exhibit 3.1, but the results don't drive decisions as often as they should. The Performance Improvement Council (PIC, Exhibit 3.2) isn't identifying a lot of projects; the list of recognized opportunities for improvement (OFIs) is short. You do the annual planning calendar (Exhibit 3.3), but mostly to set the operating budget. Quality and satisfaction measures are also "discussed."

The next step for an HCO like this is expanding the multidimensional operational and strategic performance measures, Exhibit 3.4 and 3.5, respectively. Upgrade "also discussed" to negotiated goals on Joint Commission quality measures, HCAHPS scores, and worker satisfaction data. They come with benchmarks, but you also have internal "bests" that you can celebrate and use for training. Look for easy gains ("low-hanging fruit") and accept partway-to-benchmark improvements. (There's always next year.) Don't punish or criticize anybody. Just ask them how much better they can do, realistically, next year. Remember that change in process (Exhibit 3.2) is what drives improvement.

Moving away from "cost control" to "continuous improvement" ironically is the best way to increase profit margins! Answering associate questions and setting up process improvement teams (PITs) to solve recurring problems pay off in cost-per-case. "Service excellence" combined with OFIs and PITs pay off even more handsomely.

What to Do Next?

An operating unit is well below benchmark on most of its measures. It could be a clinical service line, or a critical logistic function like supplies or food service. What does the improvement plan look like?

Your coach says:

1. If it's a multi-part unit, look at the parts, and focus on the weaker ones.
2. For each weak first-line operating unit, do this:
   a. Go there and listen. Roll up your sleeves and pitch in. Listen some more.
   b. Evaluate the unit leader, using your observations and associate measures. Arrange coaching, training, or retraining as indicated.
   c. With the unit leader, rank order the OFIs, first in terms of "easiest."
   d. Set up PITs to do the easiest, remembering that each PIT has two purposes: improve performance and teach the membership.
   e. Re-evaluate the OFIs, in terms of "most important to long-run success," and think about how to address the top priorities.
   f. Agree upon some realistic improvement goals based on the PITs, achieve them, and celebrate.
   g. Repeat.

HOW IS THE EXCELLENT INFRASTRUCTURE DIFFERENT?

All HCOs have an operational infrastructure. It's the set of mechanisms—agreements, contracts, plans, rules, committees, accountability hierarchy—by which the parts are related to the whole. It complements the culture and allows decisions to be made and implemented. Excellent HCOs make their infrastructure more reliable, faster, and more effective. They have rebuilt the traditional static HCO infrastructure to support change; change is a way of life. The core of change is Identify—Analyze—Test—Evaluate (or if you prefer, Plan—Do—Check—Act).

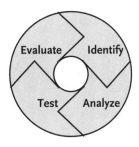

The excellent operational infrastructure:

- supports continuous improvement with measures, benchmarks, and process analysis;
- has each unit set and achieve improvement goals;
- provides the information for all daily activity and for pursuing OFIs;
- establishes the correct size for all units; and
- surveys the environment for shifts in stakeholder needs, technology, and competitive position.

An excellent infrastructure has five service functions and its own review and improvement function, as shown in Exhibit 3.1. It involves all the logistic and strategic support activities described in Chapters 10 through 15. It is managed by the senior management team. The critical rule for the infrastructure is that it fully meets all its customer needs. Effectiveness comes before efficiency; the customer service benchmarks are more important than the cost benchmarks.

An executive at a high-performing HCO might say, "We do all the parts of all the functions. We do them promptly. We do them effectively. We study how to do them even better." If she

Exhibit 3.1 Infrastructure Functions Supporting Excellence

Function	Intent	Implementation	Examples
Continuous improvement	Improve measured performance. Reach decisions in a timely and coordinated fashion.	PITs develop improved processes, guided by a PIC, which coordinates and integrates improvements. PITs and goal-setting follow a quarterly and annual calendar.	The annual goal-setting and budgeting activity proceeds according to a pre-arranged timetable initiated and finished by governing board action. PITs are scheduled to complete their work in time to coordinate with budget deadlines.
Accountability, coordination, and integration	Establish explicit expectations of every team.	Expectations and accountability are established and integrated in the annual goal-setting process.	Ninety-day plans are used to ensure reaching agreed-upon goals. HCO organizes caregiving teams into service lines and ensures that effective clinical support services are available.
Knowledge management	Provide prompt, complete, reliable information for any associate's or team's purpose.	Strong clinical and business information systems, widespread access, and a culture of communication. Training for repetitive tasks, "just-in-time" training for arising tasks.	Automated patient record and access to clinical information. E-mail and an internal website. Readily accessible "data warehouse" with current performance, trends, goals, and benchmarks.

Exhibit 3.1 *Continued*

Function	Intent	Implementation	Examples
Planning	Forecast patient needs to plan staffing and facilities.	Epidemiologic planning model establishes the size of all clinical units.	Quantified plans for services, facilities, and personnel reflect trends in community need.
Boundary-spanning and corporate design	Monitor all external stakeholder groups to identify changes in their needs/desires. Provide an integrated array that optimally meets community needs.	Governing board members, senior executives, and other managers solicit stakeholder perspectives and describe HCO opportunities. Ongoing market analysis identifies trends and stakeholder needs. Subsidiaries, joint ventures, and strategic partnerships support a broad scope of healthcare activities.	Board members selected on record of effective community service. Senior managers participate in community services for education, housing, etc. and monitor state and national developments potentially affecting the HCO. HCO includes primary and continuing care services, forms joint ventures and mergers with medical staff and other HCOs.
Improving the operational infrastructure	Improve the operational and strategic foundations.	Sessions of the governing board and senior management meetings are devoted to review of infrastructure effectiveness measures, identification of OFIs, and development of improvements.	Annual goal-setting process improved, additional performance measures installed and benchmarked. Expanded strategic protection. Expanded analytic and training support for PITs.

were particularly candid, she would add, "And there are no exceptions. No back doors. No special deals. Our infrastructure rules are 'the book,' and we go by the book."

HOW DOES INFRASTRUCTURE SUPPORT CONTINUOUS IMPROVEMENT?

The infrastructure must imbed the improvement process, the cycle of identify/analyze/test/evaluate, into the routine of the organization. The process is shown in Exhibit 3.2. It occurs constantly. Dozens of PITs are at work in an excellent HCO. The smaller ones, working within their own team, are not even counted. The larger ones are supervised by the Performance Improvement Council (PIC), an expanded version of the senior management team.

The search for OFIs must be ongoing; the PITs must make steady progress; PIT findings must be implemented; and expected results must be included in the next year's goals. The infrastructure for this has three major parts: an annual planning calendar, an internal consulting resource, and a process for conflict resolution.

Calendar for Annual Planning

Excellent HCOs maintain their timeliness with an explicit calendar tracking their fiscal year, as shown in Exhibit 3.3. Adhering to the calendar is principally the job of the senior management, as shown by their involvement throughout Exhibit 3.3.

- At step 1, the board's task is to balance customer and associate needs, establishing organization-wide goals that promote excellence but are realistically achievable.

Exhibit 3.2 Process Improvement: Changing OFIs to Improved Performance

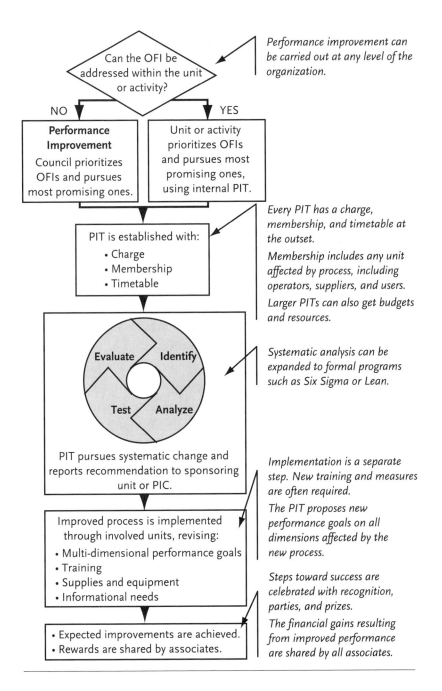

Can the OFI be addressed within the unit or activity?

Performance improvement can be carried out at any level of the organization.

NO → **Performance Improvement** Council prioritizes OFIs and pursues most promising ones.

YES → Unit or activity prioritizes OFIs and pursues most promising ones, using internal PIT.

PIT is established with:
- Charge
- Membership
- Timetable

Every PIT has a charge, membership, and timetable at the outset.

Membership includes any unit affected by process, including operators, suppliers, and users.

Larger PITs can also get budgets and resources.

Evaluate / Identify / Test / Analyze

Systematic analysis can be expanded to formal programs such as Six Sigma or Lean.

PIT pursues systematic change and reports recommendation to sponsoring unit or PIC.

Implementation is a separate step. New training and measures are often required.

Improved process is implemented through involved units, revising:
- Multi-dimensional performance goals
- Training
- Supplies and equipment
- Informational needs

The PIT proposes new performance goals on all dimensions affected by the new process.

- Expected improvements are achieved.
- Rewards are shared by associates.

Steps toward success are celebrated with recognition, parties, and prizes.

The financial gains resulting from improved performance are shared by all associates.

- At steps 2, 3, and 4, the senior management team negotiates repeatedly with division leaders who in turn work with unit managers, translating the board's strategic goals to operational goals for every unit.
- At step 5, the operational goals are coordinated and integrated. At the end of step 5, consensus is reached on the goals at all levels, and they are summarized in "dashboards," or scorecards.
- At step 6, PITs design new processes to address OFIs. The improvements they devise allow the board to raise the strategic goals in the next annual round, driving continuous improvement.

Internal Consulting

Each PIT, large or small, has a charge, a specified membership, and a timetable. PITs involving only a single unit can be informal, but might still seek technical help. Those coordinated by the PIC usually have two kinds of technical assistance from internal consulting—meeting management and systems analysis. Meeting management helps the PIT run meetings expeditiously, hear perspectives fairly, clarify positions, and get done on time. Systems analysis includes fact-finding, data collection and analysis, and formal approaches like Lean, Six Sigma, or Toyota Production System. The consultants' roles are detailed in Chapters 14 and 15.

Conflict Resolution

Conflicts, defensiveness, and denial can be anticipated in the PIT process. These are best handled in private sessions where emotions as well as facts can be explored, alternatives investigated, and accommodations made. The calendar is an essential part of conflict resolution. It establishes a deadline. Many serious conflicts will test that deadline. It is the governing board's job to hold

Exhibit 3.3 Annual Planning Calendar

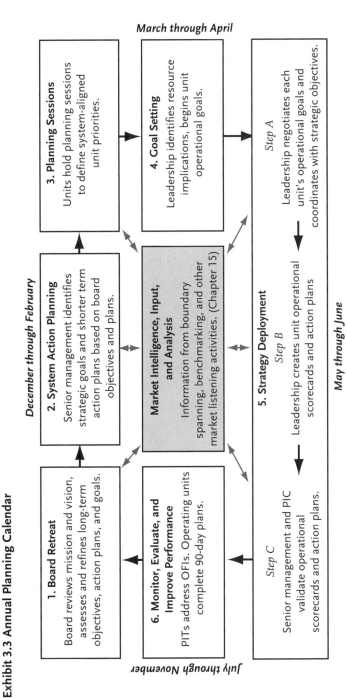

March through April

3. Planning Sessions
Units hold planning sessions to define system-aligned unit priorities.

4. Goal Setting
Leadership identifies resource implications, begins unit operational goals.

Step A
Leadership negotiates each unit's operational goals and coordinates with strategic objectives.

December through February

2. System Action Planning
Senior management identifies strategic goals and shorter term action plans based on board objectives and plans.

Market Intelligence, Input, and Analysis
Information from boundary spanning, benchmarking, and other market listening activities. (Chapter 15)

5. Strategy Deployment
Step B
Leadership creates unit operational scorecards and action plans

May through June

1. Board Retreat
Board reviews mission and vision, assesses and refines long-term objectives, action plans, and goals.

6. Monitor, Evaluate, and Improve Performance
PITs address OFIs. Operating units complete 90-day plans.

Step C
Senior management and PIC validate operational scorecards and action plans.

July through November

Adapted from Mercy Health Services MBNQA Application, p. 7.
"Leadership" is all management associates.
Note that the Market Intelligence activity is ongoing, although it is emphasized at the board's annual retreat, Step 1.

to it judiciously. That action rules out foot-dragging, red herrings, and obfuscation as strategies to protect limited interests. The culture reinforces the board's action. Listening has occurred, facts have been gathered and tested, the opinions of colleagues established. The case is won or lost, and continued objection will be fruitless and painful.

HOW IS IMPROVEMENT ROLLED OUT TO OPERATING UNITS?

Accountability

Excellent HCOs using evidence-based management have moved substantially beyond the traditional pyramid "table of organization." They retain an accountability hierarchy to negotiate goals and monitor performance. The goals and the performance are quantified, making expectations explicit.

The general template for operational measures is shown in Exhibit 3.4. This template is used throughout *Reaching Excellence* and is shown with specific measures in all chapters 4 to 15.

At the highest organization levels (service lines and the governing board) the array of information is expanded to include financial data and the measures are aggregated to the enterprise level. The template is shown in Exhibit 3.5, and a real example is shown in Exhibit 4.1.

Quantitative measures and goals make the HCO's mission and each unit's contribution explicit. They prove the improvement, justify the celebrations and bonuses, and identify the OFIs. At the same time, the transformational culture emphasizes a much more flexible approach with multiple lines of communication. The HCO's leadership team, including managers at every level, is expected to seek help from other units of the organization and to provide help when it is requested. The combination ensures that each team has a prescribed purpose, a responsive system for

Exhibit 3.4 Operational Performance Measures for Individual Teams and Activities

Input Oriented	Output Oriented
Demand	*Output/Productivity*
Requests for service	Counts of services rendered
Market share	Productivity (resources/treatment
Appropriateness of	or service)
demand	*Quality*
Unmet need	Clinical outcomes
Demand logistics	Procedural quality
Demand errors	Structural quality
Cost/Resources	*Customer Satisfaction*
Physical counts	Patients
Costs	Referring physicians
Resource condition	Other customers
Human Resources	
Supply	
Development	
Satisfaction	
Loyalty	

addressing unmet needs, and a path for negotiating improved goals.

Corporate Design

The high-performing models for *Reaching Excellence* often operate multi-site, multi-purpose systems. They are acquiring or joint-venturing with medical practices and non-acute services. They have

Exhibit 3.5 Strategic Performance Measures for the HCO Enterprise

Dimension	Major Concepts	Healthcare Examples
Financial performance	Ability to acquire, husband, and effectively reinvest essential resources	Profit and cash flow Days cash on hand Credit rating and financial structure
Internal operations, including quality and safety	Ability to provide competitive service Quality, efficiency, safety, and availability of service	Unit cost of care Measures of safety and quality of care Processes and outcomes of care Timeliness of service
Market performance and customer satisfaction	Reflects all aspects of relationship to customers	Market share Patient and family satisfaction Measures of access for disadvantaged groups
Associate satisfaction and ability to adapt and improve	Ability to attract and retain an effective associate group Learning and motivation of workforce Response to change in technology, customer attitudes, and economic environment	Physician and employee satisfaction Associate safety and retention Training program participation and skill development Availability of emerging methods of care Trends in service and market performance Ability to implement changes in timely fashion

extended their influence through consortia and partnerships with private, charitable, and government organizations that share components of the overall mission. Many also include their own healthcare financing mechanisms. The emerging corporate design includes a parent corporation, wholly owned subsidiaries, partially owned joint ventures, and long-term strategic partnership contracts without ownership. It is increasingly both vertically and horizontally integrated. The change-oriented infrastructure is extended to all of these arrangements. It is a major asset that makes the HCO attractive as a partner or an owner.

HOW CAN OUR HCO PROCESS A THOUSAND PERFORMANCE MEASURES?

Knowledge—evidence—is at the core of the high-performing infrastructure. Measuring all the dimensions required for exhibits 3.4 and 3.5 and helping each unit reach its goals require a new level of knowledge management. Poudre Valley Health System (PVHS), the 2008 healthcare Malcolm Baldrige National Quality Award (MBNQA) recipient, explains what's involved:

> PVHS' ability to meet and exceed the expectations of quality care, prompt service, and friendly staff is dependent upon the timely availability of information for the workforce, suppliers, partners, collaborators, patients, and the community. To optimize the flow of accurate, real-time information, PVHS has established a secure, user-friendly network that is appropriately accessible to all stakeholders, regardless of geography or time of day. In this network . . . the central repository [has] associated content-specific functions such as:
>
> - **Clinical Information**. Electronic health records, Picture Archive and Communication System (PACS), lab results, poison control, [automated pharmaceutical dispensing and medication reconciliation].
> - **Physician Information Center (Provider LINK)**. Clinical information (see above); subscription-based online resources, such as MD Consult, CINAHL, and online medical journals.
> - **Decision Support.** [Key Performance Indicator] reports; electronic data interchanges (automatic supply tracking, ordering, and billing with nearly 100 percent of PVHS vendors); Information Center (service utilization, patient demographics, market trends).

- **Financial Information.** Patient billing, payroll, accounts receivable, revenue cycle management
- **Employee Information Center.** Patient census (by unit or outpatient department); bed management (number of patients by unit/facility and admission/discharge projections); time clock; due dates for mandatory annual learning test, tuberculosis testing, performance reviews, time clock entries, pay stub, and benefits; performance reviews; balanced scorecard and quality data; patient satisfaction data; Medline; policies/procedures; forms; calendars; job postings; directories.
- **Patient Information Center.** GetWell Network, educational materials, gift shop, newborn photo gallery, and health resources such as a diabetes management tool and a database for identifying potential drug interactions.[1]

"Decision Support" and PVHS's "Key Performance Indicators" implement the templates, exhibits 3.4 and 3.5. The other five categories are "just-in-time" resources supporting daily activity but also providing help for PITs and units wrestling with goal achievement. An HCO moving to excellence must invest systematically in all these areas, improving them simultaneously with other operating unit needs. The plan for doing this is in Chapter 10. Knowledge management elements that are critical to the infrastructure include benchmarking, standardizing measures, training, and auditing.

Benchmarking

For every activity in an HCO like PVHS there is a best practice, the process that generates the best results. The performance achieved by best practice is the benchmark. Most HCOs start

---

[1]Poudre Valley Health System. 2008. Malcolm Baldrige National Quality Award Application. [Online information; retrieved 6/17/09.] www.baldrige.nist.gov/ PDF_files/2008_Poudre_Valley_Application_Summary.pdf, pp. 17–18.

benchmarking locally, expand it to national comparisons, and at PVHS's level seek "world class."

No HCO achieves benchmark for every measure. Even Baldrige recipients have OFIs. The PIC's job is often not to *achieve* benchmarks; it's to *move toward* benchmarks. Rome was not built in a day; it is wiser to set a realistic goal, make it, and celebrate than to over-reach, fail, and frustrate.

Standardizing Measures

Benchmarking requires uniform measures. Realistic goals require realistic measures. High-performing HCOs use a measurement review committee that assists in the development and testing of new measures. The committee emphasizes nationally defined measures as a priority, both because these definitions are rigorously developed and tested and because national standardization is essential for benchmarking. When unique measures must be developed or national measures adjusted for local conditions, the committee provides expert assistance.

Training and Open Access

The infrastructure for high performance is not intuitive, it's learned. High-performing HCOs are distinguished by their commitment to training, 80 to more than 100 hours a year per full-time associate, about twice the average investment.[2] Just-in-time training and self-training are commonplace. Coaching a new manager and helping a PIT chairperson manage a meeting are just-in-time examples. (*Reaching Excellence* can be used both in scheduled and just-in-time applications. Professional managers

---

[2]Griffith, J. R. 2009. "Finding the Frontier of Hospital Management." *Journal of Healthcare Management* 54 (1): 59–72.

master its content to construct effective systems. They and others refer to it to answer specific questions.)

High-performing HCOs deliberately pursue a strategy of broad access to the system. Privacy and competitive requirements are met, but beyond them, the strategy is to make information available. Access is speeded by electronic records and search engines. PVHS notes that it also communicates "through newsletters, reports, bulletin boards, posters, mailings, media, and [other] approaches."[3] Open access enhances empowerment, speeds communication, and reduces errors. Under this strategy, much information becomes public, or nearly so. The dangers cited against broad access—competitors, lawsuits, misinterpretations—have not proven to be significant.

Auditing

Audits serve two important purposes. They prevent fraud and they validate measures. High-performing HCOs have extended the internal audit activity to all dimensions of the operational and strategic scorecards and strengthened the audit activity to Sarbanes-Oxley criteria (see Is Auditing an 'Onstage' Function? in Chapter 13). The result is not so much reduced losses as increased assurance. "We don't argue about the measures anymore."

WHAT IS THE RIGHT SIZE FOR AN OPERATING UNIT?

A unit that's too small fails to meet demand. One that's too big has high costs and can have quality problems. To provide effective size, high-performing HCOs use an epidemiologic planning

---

[3]Poudre Valley Health System. 2008. Malcolm Baldrige National Quality Award Application, p. 18.

model, a tool that forecasts the number of patients requiring a specific service. The elements of the model are shown in Exhibit 3.6.

The epidemiologic planning model is implemented by purchasing access to a sophisticated computerized analysis that combines population forecasts and usage data from a variety of national sources and applies them to local areas. The resulting projections are translated to actual personnel and facility forecasts by internal or external consultants who negotiate the personnel and facilities parameters with local associates. The size of many support services, like parking and human resources, is driven by the aggregate forecast of clinical services. The process is described further in Chapter 14. The epidemiologic planning model is essential to virtually every service and is referenced in all the following chapters.

The final decision on the size of clinical services is reserved for the governing board. Senior management is responsible for negotiating a recommendation that is acceptable both to the associates involved in the service and the board.

HOW DOES OUR HCO KEEP ON TRACK WITH ITS STAKEHOLDERS?

Rank ordering the OFIs and setting the annual goals require an ongoing system of listening and negotiation with customers. The program that helps Sharp HealthCare relate to the San Diego community is an example. Sharp, a 2007 recipient of the MBNQA, claims its "involvement in San Diego's well-being is comprehensive."

- When key community health issues or new health threats are identified, Sharp collaborates with appropriate public officials for safe, evidence-based, patient-centered, timely, efficient, and equitable resolution.
- Sharp's leaders serve as board members on many community organizations.

Exhibit 3.6 Elements of the Epidemiologic Planning Model

For any specific clinical service:

Question	Solution	Example
What population will use the service?	People who live in small geographic areas. The population of these areas is measured and forecast by the U.S. Census Bureau.	Births for Ann Arbor, Michigan, and surrounding areas
What part of that population is at risk for the service?	The risk of a disease is dependent on age, genetics, income, and lifestyle. These factors are used to forecast demand.	Births are a function of the number of females by age and certain socio-economic characteristics.
What part of the population at risk will select our service?	Historical data and surveys estimate the fraction of those with the disease seeking care from our team (market share).	Women around Ann Arbor choose between two obstetrics services. Home deliveries and travel to other services are rare.
How many specialized people will we need to meet this demand?	Protocols, historical data, and benchmarks show the number of patients an individual provider can successfully treat.	Each of the OB services must establish the numbers of obstetricians, family practitioners, midwives, registered nurses, and other caregivers required.
How big a facility will we need to meet this demand?	History, benchmarks, and simulation models show how many rooms and specialized facilities will be required.	The 2012 University of Michigan obstetrical delivery service will have "50 single room maternity care beds in the Birth Center."*

*http://www.med.umich.edu/mott/touch/new_facts.html [Online information; retrieved 4/21/09].

- Sharp's comprehensive environmental, health, and safety management program, including emergency/disaster management, ensures a safe and secure environment for customers/partners.
- Staff and leaders present a strong showing of support and participation each year in community fundraisers.
- Sharp hosts many free community preventive health offerings, such as flu shots, lectures, and screenings.
- Sharp offers the Weight Management Health Education program, providing health maintenance to employers and employees and free, weekly programs to the community.
- Managers are encouraged to donate a minimum of 22,000 collective hours annually to community service.[4]

HOW DO WE IMPROVE THE INFRASTRUCTURE?

The senior leadership team must apply continuous improvement to the infrastructure itself. Many qualitative indicators arise from various listening activities and unexpected events. Examples are shown in Exhibit 3.7. "Systematic listening," suggested several times in the exhibit, includes logs or written reports of noteworthy findings. The logs are aggregated and critically reviewed. Quantitative indicators, shown in Exhibit 3.8, should be improving. Members of the PIC can individually identify and rank order infrastructure OFIs. Their written reports can be aggregated and consensus reached using nominal group technique. Using several perspectives generates a more objective and thorough evaluation.

The interpretation of infrastructure measures is not as straightforward as most operational and strategic measures. Qualitative

---

[4]Sharp HealthCare. 2007. Malcolm Baldrige National Quality Award Application [Online information; retrieved 12/16/08.] www.baldrige.nist.gov/Contacts_Profiles.htm, Preface, p. 6.

Exhibit 3.7 Qualitative Indicators of Infrastructure OFIs

Function	Qualitative Indicators	Sources
Continuous improvement	Difficulty in negotiating goals Complaints about PITs or timetable Critical shortfalls from benchmark	Minutes and observations of PIC participants Boundary-spanning
Accountability and organization design	Effectiveness of PITs Customer and associate complaints or service concerns Effective adoption of new technology	Logs of systematic listening and unanticipated events Associate and stakeholder comments Consultants' advice and record of other HCOs
Knowledge management	Associate complaints or concerns Success of new hires and promotions Terminal interview comments	Systematic listening and comments of associate stakeholders Individual interviews and personal evaluations
Planning	Appearance and "feel" are neither overcrowded nor empty Requests for service expansion Competitive services and equipment	Minutes and observations of PIC participants Customer and associate comments
Boundary-spanning	Stated satisfaction of major customer stakeholders Competitor activities Activities of excellent HCOs in other communities Changes in healthcare financing, technology Changes in local employment, attitudes, or civic commitments	Systematic listening and comments of customer stakeholder leadership Published and suspected actions of competitors Published reports and awards Consultants' reports Government legislation and regulation Reports from literature, trade and professional associations

information is relatively more important. The full array of opportunities must be carefully explored to establish the right goals. The key questions for evaluation are:

1. Is the HCO moving in the correct long-term direction? Has the overall progress been sufficient?
2. Is progress uniformly deployed across the HCO?
3. What are the most important OFIs and improvement goals?

The evaluation is usually carried out by both the governing board and senior leadership.

WHAT ARE THE WEAK LINKS OR RISK FACTORS FOR THE MODEL?

So far, none of the documented implementations has reported difficulties that caused them to question the model, and they are strongly committed to pursuing it further. A review of the weak links must therefore be hypothetical, but careful consideration suggests the following areas.

1. Physician and nurse relations are crucial to the culture and to overall success.
2. Changes in the payment system make the model more important.
3. Unrealistic governing board demands could threaten the model.
4. Implementation failure could threaten the model.
5. Evidence of lack of sincere commitment to the mission could threaten the model.

These factors are all monitored closely in the systems described above.

Exhibit 3.8 Performance Measures for Infrastructure Functions

Function	Infrastructure Concept	Measures	Source	Examples
Continuous improvement	Goal achievement	Percent of goals met	Enterprise information system	Strategic measures, Exhibit 3.5
	Goal improvement	MBNQA Score	Outside consultants	
Organization design	Uniformity of performance	Market share	Surveys of market share	Patients leaving area for care
	Extent of service	Efficiency of care	Cost per case and length of stay	Case-mix adjusted cost per case
	Competitor relations	Per capita cost of care	Analysis of trends, and percent of benchmark for operational and strategic measures	Dartmouth Atlas* cost and use per capita
		Variation in internal performance improvement		Unit(s) not progressing toward benchmark
		Unmet or delayed demand		Undersized unit with service delays
				Oversized unit with excess capacity
				Competitor growth

Exhibit 3.8 Continued

Function	Infrastructure Concept	Measures	Source	Examples
Knowledge management	Goal improvement	System availability, "hits"	Information system	"Down time" for 24/7 systems
		Percent of goals achieved	Analysis of performance	Number of "90-day correction plans"
		User satisfaction surveys	Surveys	Budget delivered on time
		Delays in annual planning process	Annual planning activity	

Continued

Exhibit 3.8 Continued

Function	Infrastructure Concept	Measures	Source	Examples
Boundary-spanning	Maximizing external stakeholder satisfaction	Trends and variations in satisfaction surveys	Ongoing patient surveys	Surveys of employers and potential patients
		Counts of unanticipated events	Ad hoc surveys of other stakeholders	Profit and funds available for investment
		Financial performance	Records of complaints and incidents	Bond rating
		Quality-of-care measures	Financial reports	Global patient satisfaction scores
		Community health measures	Medical records	Adverse patient care events
			Community health surveys	Percent of community immunized
				Percent of community with premature loss of life or function
Sustaining and improving	Continuous improvement	Board scores	Board self-evaluation	Percent of board stating "complete satisfaction"
		Outside audits	Auditor reports	Joint Commission deficiencies

*The Dartmouth Atlas of Hospital Use, a web-based, small-area reporting system, provides estimates of cost per capita and hospital days per capita from Medicare data. See http://www.dartmouthatlas.org/ [Online information; retrieved 4/15/09].

SUGGESTED READINGS

Butler, G., and C. Caldwell. 2008. *What Top-Performing Healthcare Organizations Know: 7 Proven Steps for Accelerating and Achieving Change.* Chicago: Health Administration Press.

Collins, J. C. 2009. *How the Mighty Fall . . . and Why Some Companies Never Give In.* New York: HarperCollins.

Malcolm Baldrige National Quality Program. 2009. "Health Care Criteria for Performance Excellence." [Online information; retrieved 3/11/09.] www.baldrige.nist.gov/ PDF_files/2009_2010_HealthCare_Criteria.pdf.

Pfeffer, J., and R. I. Sutton. 2006. *Hard Facts, Dangerous Half-Truths, and Total Nonsense: Profiting from Evidence-Based Management.* Boston: Harvard Business School Press.

Chapter 4   In a Few Words . . .

The governing board implements the strategic direction through five specific activities. It monitors and improves its own performance in a sixth:

1. Select and work with the CEO
2. Establish the mission, vision, and values
3. Approve strategies and an annual budget to implement the mission
4. Maintain the quality of care
5. Monitor results for compliance to goals, laws, and regulation
6. Continuously improve the governance function

Board performance is measured by HCO performance, using the strategic scorecard and the board's own systematic review.

The critical issue is accomplishing the agenda in a prudent and effective manner. The solution is an active, committed board, carefully and extensively complemented by effective management and an extensive network of committees and listening activities.

Boards succeed at the critical decisions because they follow carefully designed processes for selecting and educating members, managing their agenda, and improving their own performance.

Creating Excellent Governance

Is This Your Hospital?

Your governing board is at least "pretty good." They're sincere, hard-working community leaders who take their roles for prudence and trust seriously. Your HCO provides a "pretty good" board orientation, but it tends to focus on history, not board processes. You have a strategic scorecard, and you'll improve it a little next year. Checking against Exhibit 4.2, though, there's at least one opportunity for improvement (OFI) for each of the 10 items.

The solution is multi-step, but not hard, given a capable chair.

1. Share your findings with the chair. Point out where the OFIs are and stress the potential results in terms of board performance and board satisfaction:

   a. The board could more reliably make the right decisions.
   b. It could protect itself against legal action and stakeholder complaint.
   c. It would send a strong signal to rest of the associates.

2. Propose a board education program: a guest, either a knowledgeable consultant or a CEO or board chair from a non-competing, high-performing HCO.

---

3. Suggest an expanded nominations committee or an ad hoc committee built around the board's most respected leaders to serve as a process improvement team (PIT) on board processes and a prototype governance committee.

The key to success is having all board members understand the goals: better decisions, better legal protection, clearer signals to the associates.

What to Do Next?

Several recurring board OFIs have time-tested solutions. Here's what your coach says:

- Too many members: Limit terms. Set up an honorific board and "promote" members to it without replacement on the governing board.
- Too much time on the wrong problems: Build the committee structure and the consent agenda. Push the micromanagement down into focused sub-committees.
- Non-performing members: An officer or two takes the subject to lunch, expresses the concerns, and asks what can be done about them. Also make re-appointment less than automatic. Negotiate an "honorable discharge."
- Control freaks: Get them a coach. Go over the agenda in advance with them. Show them the record. Put them on committees and sub-committees, such as finance and audit, where their scrutiny will probably help and they can scrutinize without taking everyone's time.
- Self-interest or conflict of interest: Ask your legal counsel to provide an educational session on Exhibit 4.2, Item 6, and implement the self-evaluation, Item 5. Another lunch may be in order.

WHAT IS EXCELLENT GOVERNANCE?

The "trust" in "trustee" is the fiduciary obligation to the community that owns the HCO:

> **to create and maintain foundations for relationships among the stakeholders that identify and implement their wishes as effectively as possible.**

In excellent HCOs, excellent governance is achieved by a carefully structured system that expects six functions from the board:

1. Employing and evaluating (or if necessary, replacing) the CEO and encouraging and supporting the senior leadership team.
2. Identifying and implementing the mission and the strategic direction.
3. Guiding the annual plans for improvement.
4. Maintaining clinical excellence.
5. Monitoring and rewarding progress toward excellence.
6. Continuously improving the board's own effectiveness.

Like other parts of modern healthcare, these are complex functions, carried out by sophisticated people. The excellent board follows clear procedures and a formal calendar. It expects a significant contribution of time from its members, who are drawn from the community's "best and brightest." It relies on management to provide the major part of the knowledge resources for those functions, including training for board members. Relations with the CEO and senior management are the first function because none of the other five can be completed without them. Management's obligations—the things that must be done to guide and implement the board's decisions—are in the other chapters of *Reaching Excellence*. Conceptually, it is the board's role to identify excellence. Management's role is both to provide much of the knowledge required to identify excellence and to deliver what the board has identified.

Performance is measured, benchmarked, and improved in governance as in all areas. The central measure of board performance is the HCO's strategic scorecard. An example, from Saint Luke's Hospital in Kansas City, Missouri, is shown in Exhibit 4.1. The board is doing a good job when these measures are improving toward benchmark.

Excellent boards now operate under carefully constructed procedures, as shown in Exhibit 4.2. These are designed to allow many voices to be heard, maintain objectivity and balance, and promote wise consensus. Operating as Exhibit 4.2 suggests, most meetings are focused on a single issue or a few related issues that are thoroughly documented by management and presented to the board as alternatives for resolution. Part of the board's and management's skill is in identifying the critical elements. Many important decisions are simply presented as the "consent agenda," which is normally passed without discussion but allows any member to request debate if she feels that it is necessary.

IS THERE ANOTHER GOOD WAY TO DO GOVERNANCE?

In a word, no. There are countless other ways to do governance, but none has documented long-term success. Most do not even document short-term success; they simply prove that mediocrity is always possible. The paths to failure are also uncountable, but weaker HCOs fall prey to one or both of two major dangers:

1. They cannot achieve consensus, fail to meet their calendar deadlines, and bring improvement to a standstill. As a result, the HCO loses the forward momentum that leads to excellence.
2. They fail to balance stakeholder needs. One group of stakeholders (it can be a part of the community population, a cabal of business leaders, parts of the medical staff, unions,

Exhibit 4.1 Saint Luke's Hospital Balanced Scorecard

Saint Luke's Hospital Scorecard

Scoring Criteria 2010

	Key Measures	Bench-mark	Adj. Score	+4 / 9	+3 / 8	+2 / 7	+1 / 6	Goal / 5	-1 / 4	-2 / 3	-3 / 2	-4 / 1	Raw Score
PEOPLE	Retention												
	RN Vacancy Rate												
	Employee Satisfaction**												
	Diversity												
CLINICAL & ADMINISTRATIVE QUALITY	Inpatient Clinical Care Index												
	Appropriate Care Measure (ACM) Index												
	Order Set Utilization Index												
	eICU Index												
	Outpatient Clinical Care Index												
	Patient Safety Index												
	Operational Index												
	Infection Control Index												
	Medical Staff Clinical Indicator Index												
CUSTOMER SATISFACTION	Would Recommend (HCAHPS)												
	Patient Loyalty - SLHS "Would Recommend" 5's only												
	Timeliness of Care and Service												
	Responsiveness to Patient Needs												
	Aver ER Wait time - Home Disposition (Tracking BRD)												
	Student Education Index												
GROWTH & DEVELOPMENT	Eligible IP Market Share (Primary/Secondary)												
	Eligible IP Market Share - Strategic Product Lines												
	Profitable Eligible IP Market Share (Primary Only)												
	OP Surgeries - Count												
	Unsuccessful ER to ER Transfers Not Meeting Criteria												
	Days to Budget												
	Research Index												
FINANCIAL	Operating Margin												
	Operating Cash Flow												
	Days Cash on Hand												
	Net Days in Accounts Receivable (IP/OP)												
	Patient Volume (revenue % to budget)												
	Realization Rate vs Budget												

Notes within scoring columns: Scores at this level will be flagged blue. / Scores in the green range will be flagged in green. / Scores at this level will be flagged in yellow. / Scores at this level will be flagged in blue.

** Indicates annual measure.

Exceeding Goal / Goal / Moderate / Risk		2010 Overall Score	1 Qtr	2 Qtr	3 Qtr	4 Qtr	Overall Score / Goal / Stretch

For current performance to be scored greater than Level 1, the current performance value must meet or exceed the scoring criteria within a Level.

For FINANCIAL: Scoring ranges based on agency ratings

Note: The scoring criteria was modified in 2006: The scoring range changed from a 10-tier range to a 9-tier range, and the color coding for meeting goal was expanded to accommodate common cause variation.

or senior management) dominates the decision process, with the result that other stakeholders transfer their loyalties elsewhere.

Exhibit 4.2 Ten Measures of Board Effectiveness

1. Meeting legal requirements	Bond rating agencies include a "due diligence" review of the organization's compliance with all outstanding legal obligations; the board, at a minimum, should always require that one of its committees have access to all such due diligence reports and any responses from senior management.
2. Compliance orientation	Corporate compliance is a process of honest self-scrutiny, often involving objective third-party evaluators. When done properly, it produces an attorney-client privileged report that the board of directors or an appropriate board committee can study in depth; they should also monitor steps taken in response to the report. Boards should insist that senior management develop a corporate compliance mentality, in which legal shortcomings are routinely defined, identified, analyzed, and corrected. A formal compliance program reduces legal risks and constitutes another best practice of good governance.
3. Continuing governance education (CGE)	The board chair, the CEO, and the governance committee chair should together take the lead in ensuring meaningful continuing governance education (CGE) for the entire board, not just its new members. Every board should have a formal and informal CGE calendar for each year, supplemented with discussions led by individual board members after their attendance at CGE events.
4. Use of dashboards	Dashboards (e.g., Saint Luke's strategic scorecard, Exhibit 4.1) help boards realize that policy decisions should result in performance improvements. Appropriate and regular use of dashboards will build governance confidence and will distinguish those boards from boards not using such governance best practices.

Exhibit 4.2 *Continued*

5. Agenda practice	Some form of board self-evaluation and executive session should occur at each board meeting. Good practice encourages questions, seeks balanced presentations, and makes a deliberate effort not to disparage any good-faith question.
6. Conflicts of interest*	Conflicts of interest should be announced at every meeting. "If board members will just remember three simple rules about conflicts of interest, they will generally want to do the right things. a. Undisclosed conflicts are, by definition, not 'in good faith,' which has the legal effect of nullifying all the directors' statutory immunities. b. Undisclosed conflicts can, since 1996, produce substantial federal excise taxes on affected individuals who are corporate insiders and who obtain excess benefits from their organizations. c. An apparent, but not real, conflict can cause almost as much trouble as a real one in terms of public embarrassment for individuals and [not-for-profit] boards."
7. Corporate governance committee	The committee should meet regularly throughout the year; seek and nominate appropriate new members; review all outside reports and board effectiveness materials, plans, and continuing education; propose new measures, procedures, and bylaws as indicated; and investigate violations of confidentiality and conflict-of-interest policies.
8. Voluntary Sarbanes-Oxley compliance	The landmark Sarbanes-Oxley Act does not apply to not-for-profit organizations except as to whistleblower protection. But its rationales do apply. Governance committees should study the act and recommend such easily identifiable steps as CEO and CFO certification of financial statements and clarification of who should and should not serve on the board and various committees.

Exhibit 4.2 *Continued*

9. CEO evaluation   CEO evaluation is best coordinated through a board committee but all members of the board should be invited expressly to participate. The evaluation should relate to board-established objectives and include an opportunity for open-ended comments as well as responses to specific questions. The evaluation should directly affect a year-end bonus or the next year's base compensation. The board chair should share the evaluation with the CEO in a personal meeting. The process should include both the CEO's self-evaluation and the CEO's reaction to the board's evaluation.

10. Board planning and evaluation   Each of the foregoing nine areas of conduct includes some form of planning for the institution, but no single one of them asks whether the full board is invested in helping plan the overall future of the organization.

Board self-analysis should include what all directors/trustees think about:

a. their collective tackling of the foregoing nine measurable elements in the last year,

b. the organization's prospects for the future, and

c. their individual contributions and/or misgivings about what each has done or not done for the organization.

*Conflicts of interest: real or potential personal financial benefit that may accrue from a given board decision.

SOURCE: Used with permission from Bryant, L. E., Jr., and P. D. Jacobson. 2005. "Measuring Nonprofit Health Care Governance Effectiveness: How Do You Know a Good Thing When You See It? Ten Easy Measures of Nonprofit Board Conduct." *Modern Healthcare* (Supplement), December.

Excellent HCOs are more diligent than others in guarding against these dangers. They find the resources to resolve debate and meet their calendar. They diligently and scrupulously solicit and study the full array of stakeholder needs, and as Exhibit 4.2 states, they rigorously control conflict of interest.

WHAT MAKES THIS MODEL WORK?

At first glance, the summary message is "discipline." The board must be prudent, deliberate, fair, and timely in completing its functions. The reality is more complicated. As in sports and the performing arts, discipline is mostly a matter of training and practice. What makes the model work can be summarized into four categories:

1. A transformational culture empowers stakeholders, expands knowledge, and encourages debate. An evidence-based culture makes facts the criterion for decisions around a consensus mission, vision, and values.
2. Knowledge management delivers the right facts on time to the right people.
3. The infrastructure ensures timely and effective implementation of the decisions made.
4. The board members are selected and trained for their role, and they work on improving their contribution.

The culture, knowledge management, and the infrastructure are the core tasks of management. The other chapters of *Reaching Excellence* describe how it's done. Good governance depends upon good management.

HOW ARE BOARD MEMBERS RECRUITED?

Boards are kept small, around 15 members. Members are generally expected to serve two terms of three years, meaning that two or three people are replaced each year and half the board has more than three years experience. Nominating committees seek members through a continuing search. Ongoing training helps members make the biggest possible contribution. Members should bring familiarity with the community and its diverse elements. They should be experienced in enterprise-level decision making and have the time (at least one full day per month) to devote to board duties. A record for success and a reputation of probity are important. Board members act as a whole; they do not "represent" stakeholders or constituencies. In not-for-profit HCOs they are almost always volunteers. The role of "insiders," people employed by the HCO, has been diminished. The CEO and a few physicians are often members; they are excused in the "executive sessions" in Exhibit 4.2, Item 5.

HOW ARE BOARD MEMBERS TRAINED?

While new members should bring fresh perspectives, they should not operate in ignorance of history. New-member orientation programs include tours, interviews with key personnel, review of major policies and decisions, and dialog. A typical list of subjects is shown in Exhibit 4.3. Catholic Health Initiatives, a successful HCO system operating in 20 states, mandates a three-day offsite training program for each new trustee in its member HCOs.[1]

Much learning after orientation is from practice. Well-organized boards make committee appointments carefully, allowing new members to become acquainted with the organization in

---

[1]Griffith, J. R., and K. R. White. 2003. *Thinking Forward: Six Strategies for Highly Successful Organizations*. Chicago: Health Administration Press.

Exhibit 4.3 Board Member Orientation Subjects

Mission, Role, and History of HCOs

What healthcare organizations give to the community

Difference between for-profit, not-for-profit, and government ownership

How HCOs Are Financed

Operating funds

Private insurance

Government insurance

Uninsured patients

Sources and uses of capital funds

How HCOs Strive for Excellence

Quality and safety agenda

Service lines

Empowerment and transformational management culture

Performance measurement

Continuous improvement

HCO-Physician Relations

Nature of contract between doctors and healthcare organizations

Concept of peer review

Trustee responsibilities for the medical staff

Functions of the Governing Board

Maintain management capability

Establish the mission, vision, and values

Approve the corporate strategy and annual implementation

Ensure quality and appropriate medical care

Monitor organizational performance

Continuously improve board performance

Duties of Trustees

Duty of trust

Duty of prudence

Conflict of interest

Fiduciary and compliance duties

Trustee liability

---

less demanding assignments. They fill chairs with experienced members; they use chairs and organization executives to help members learn as they serve. In addition, high performing HCOs now include educational programs in their agenda. These serve to clarify specific situations, keep the board current with national and regional trends, and provide background on complex issues.

HOW DOES THE BOARD COMPLETE ITS WORK?

The key to effective board management—getting 15 exceptionally able people to settle the business of a large corporation in a short period of time—is a combination of effective management and an extended committee structure. Only the most critical decisions actually occupy the board's time. These reach the board with a clear recommendation. Management develops the recommendations to reflect a thorough understanding of various positions and as much consensus as possible. A much larger number of issues are resolved in management committees and presented to the board for final approval. Board members can participate in these committees as indicated. The committee decisions constitute the consent agenda. A still larger number of decisions are made within board-established parameters, such as the medical staff bylaws or the annual planning goals. While there is usually an appeals process for aggrieved stakeholders, the board reviews only cases where the decision process is questionable. Questions of fact are resolved by subordinate committees.

HOW DOES THE BOARD IMPROVE ITS PERFORMANCE?

The outcomes measure of board performance is Exhibit 4.1. The process measures include:

- evaluation of the educational programs—board members should be able to say "I learned ways to do my job better";
- surveys promoting reflective review of board and personal performance; and

- an annual review session, led by the governance sub-committee.

Governance and nominating are usually combined in one committee. The committee role is to assemble the data and suggest opportunities for improvement and ways to address them.

WHAT IS THE ROLE OF HEALTH SYSTEMS?

Most large not-for-profit multi-hospital systems rely on local boards to identify and meet local stakeholder needs. Excellent systems invest heavily in training these boards and in building the culture, knowledge management, and infrastructure essential for sound governance. They monitor local board performance carefully, and reserve powers to review and if necessary change the results of any critical board decision. They should be able to improve the benchmarking of Exhibit 4.1 and provide substantial assistance on board processes. The evidence to date does not suggest that health systems have done these tasks as effectively as they could.

WHERE ARE THE WEAK LINKS?

As the board officers, members, and senior management assess and improve governance, they should look with special care at these areas, which have proven troublesome in the past.

Breaking the Tradition of Mediocrity

Identify or create by persuasion a reform cadre. Capture the nominating committee; improve nominee qualifications. Increase the education. Increase the knowledge flow. Introduce more effective alternatives to proposals under consideration. Use an executive committee, backed by an honorific larger group, to reduce the working board to effective size. Reward past service handsomely. Foundation boards and similar devices allow honor and recognition while the work is done by others.

Financial Planning

The long-range financial plan (LRFP) is a sophisticated financial forecasting model that integrates the strategic business plans and tests their reality. It is also used to identify financial needs and financing opportunities. The governing board initiates the annual planning process (Exhibit 3.3) by setting financial goals from analysis of the LRFP. The analysis itself is the job of the finance committee. Careful exploration of alternatives expands the potential for improvement and protects against future financial difficulties.

The model of transformational management and continuous improvement does not require unmanageable financial burdens. Improvements in care processes reduce the incidence of clinical complications, shortening stay and permitting higher profits. Properly carried out, the process snowballs. Further improvements increase funds for investment.

Auditing

The goal of audits is not only greater protection against fraud but also greater accuracy in reporting and greater trust about the numbers throughout the organization. Good practice now requires that all audit activities report directly to the governing board, usually through an audit committee. The audit committee selects, instructs, and receives the report of the internal auditors, external auditor, and The Joint Commission. It receives any reports from regulatory review and compliance agencies. The expectation for each of these reports is "without material departure from standard." Any other finding is an immediate OFI, to be addressed without delay.

Internal Board Members

The CEO, senior management, and clinical leaders can contribute to most board discussions. As noted in Exhibit 4.2, excellent boards excuse them routinely so the outside board members may go into executive session and converse freely.

The medical and nursing staff members on the board do not "represent" the clinical staffs. They provide clinical perspective to guide other board members.

Representation

Representation—empowerment—of all associates, including the medical staff and nursing staff, is achieved by the infrastructure and the decision processes used for process improvement teams (PITs), goal-setting, and planning. The measure of representation is in survey responses—the empowerment question can be asked directly—and listening activities. The goal is that every associate feels confident that he can change the work environment to improve mission achievement. In reality, this means that the associate knows where to turn to ask questions and get responsive answers.

A similar approach can be applied to external stakeholders. The small board is challenged both to reflect the diversity of community opinion and to complete the agenda with due diligence. The solution to those problems is extensive use of committees and sub-committees and community listening activities (see Chapter 15). Properly employed, these devices are far more effective than board seats. Ideally, any group with an agenda should be confident that its agenda is fairly heard and all reasonable responses have been made.

The result is that the board is free to represent the whole, making the decisions that advance all stakeholders' interests rather than resolving disagreements between stakeholders.

Strategic Positioning

The purpose of the focused agenda is to ensure that the board addresses its functions, but it simultaneously encourages discussion that can be completed in a less central environment. Many issues arising in board discussion are referred to standing or ad hoc committees, and within these committees to sub-committees or less formal discussion. Moving the issue away from the boardroom allows more voices to be heard, more alternatives to be explored, and more candid expressions of viewpoint. Senior management plays a critical role in this process. It identifies stakeholders with interests and brings them to the committees. It seeks best practices that demonstrate ways others have solved the issues. It painstakingly explores positions, developing the widespread understanding that is the first stage of negotiating solutions.

Over-Reaching

The board's decisions on the annual strategic goals should be carefully weighed. The goals should be as small as possible, with "stretch goals" to reflect future needs. It is easy to deal with surpassing a goal; failing to meet one can create serious difficulties. Expecting too much too fast can endanger improvement. The approach used by excellent HCOs requires training new habits that take time to install. It is founded on celebration and rewards, meaning that almost all goals are actually met and rewards are distributed. As noted in Chapter 1, substantial improvements can be reached in three years. It may not be prudent to pursue faster gains.

Due Diligence

The goal-setting process is also more fragile than meets the eye. Progress usually involves designing proposals that meet most or all stakeholder needs, and do not impair the special needs of any one group. Proposals that might generate powerful resistance are avoided. Compromise is the rule; radical reform is rare. This realism is inherent in the empowerment culture and the value of respect. The fact that HCOs using this model succeed shows that there are avenues where important progress can be made. Extensive negotiation is often necessary to find them. It takes place at all levels, from individual meetings to major committees, but rarely in the board meeting itself. Senior managers often negotiate directly to shape proposals that will gain consensus. Their skill at shaping consensus proposals and then implementing them "as advertised" is a major factor in maintaining stakeholder loyalty.

Distressed Situations

The governance chapter, like the rest of *Reaching Excellence,* assumes "pretty good," a stable, reasonably congenial and effective HCO, as its starting point. The model has been successfully applied to much less promising situations. Several steps are usually involved:

- The governing board is restructured to remove members who contributed to the failure.
- The corporate structure is revised, often by joining a healthcare system with a proven record.

- Most of senior management is replaced.
- Cost reductions necessary to achieve stable cash flows are identified and implemented.
- The new team revises the culture and infrastructure, in part by retraining the retained managers.

This approach is successful if a core of loyal, effective associates can be identified and protected, and if the new team is diligent in rebuilding. Many "turnarounds" have failed because cost reductions failed to protect a team that could do the rebuilding, and the governing board failed to recognize the need for fundamental revisions to the culture and infrastructure.

SUGGESTED READINGS

Conger, J. A. (ed.). 2009. *Boardroom Realities: Building Leaders Across Your Board.* San Francisco: Jossey-Bass.

Joshi, M. S., and B. J. Horak. 2009. *Healthcare Transformation: A Guide for the Hospital Board Member.* Chicago: American Hospital Association.

McGinn, P. 2009. *Partnership of Equals: Practical Strategies for Healthcare CEOs and Their Boards.* Chicago: Health Administration Press.

Chapter 5   In a Few Words . . .

Excellent care is care that meets or exceeds the Institute of Medicine aims—safe, effective, patient-centered, timely, efficient, and equitable. It is the core business of the HCO and the foundation that integrates all of the clinical professions. Excellence is achieved through the appropriate use and continuous improvement of protocols based on the best available clinical evidence. An excellent HCO has both patient management and functional protocols to guide clinical care, training so that its associates are skilled at implementing the protocols, and a clinical improvement plan that measures and benchmarks performance and stays current with science. Many believe it should also have strategies for improving community health. Clinical excellence is measured and benchmarked. It requires service lines and a closely integrated system of patient referral, nursing, and clinical support systems.

Foundations
of Excellent Care

Is This Your HCO?

The relationship between your HCO and its professional caregivers (doctors and nurses) is good, but it could be better.
What keeps it strong is that the caregivers (1) know what to do,
(2) know their colleagues know what to do, (3) know they are
empowered to change the work when the mission is endangered, (4) have reasonable income security, (5) have minimal
malpractice risk, and (6) have a system, including training and
technical investments, to keep up with advances in care.

Chapter 5 explains that this success is built around credentialing, protocols, planning, and training (Exhibit 5.1), making
the HCO a great place to give care. The building blocks are:

1. *Accurate diagnoses.* Only clinical professionals can do
   this critical job. They need labs, imaging, and consultation to do it right. So the HCO runs an efficient, effective and largely out-of-sight credentialing program
   (Chapter 6), with prompt, discreet intervention when
   individual caregiver performance lags. It makes its
   diagnostic support services (Chapter 8) document
   their excellent quality, reliability, and service.

2. *Protocols.* They're universal and up to date. Protocol review is ongoing. Protocol application is flexible; the interdisciplinary plan of care (IPOC) is designed to individualize care around patient need.
3. *Planning.* The array of services, whether aimed at excellence in care or community health, meets three planning goals. It ensures competitive quality, it ensures HCO financial stability, and it assures each caregiver of a competitive income.
4. *Training.* Big teams require consistently performing associates. Implementing the IPOC begins with relying on each associate to do her thing right. That's achieved with training.

What to Do Next?

The "pretty good" HCO now uses more than 100 patient management protocols, and a much larger number of functional protocols. Of course it tracks Joint Commission quality measures, and often many others. With benchmarks and unexpected event reports, these create a challenging list of clinical opportunities for improvement (OFIs). OFIs are addressed by teams, which *Reaching Excellence* calls process improvement teams (PITs).

Your coach says, "You can call them what you want, but here's the checklist of what to do to make clinical PITs effective." (It works pretty well for other PITs, too.)

1. Make sure the OFI is both material and significant. That is, most people agree that it's an important subject, and performance is two or three standard deviations below benchmark.
2. Give the PIT a charge, a membership, a timetable, and a resources commitment at the outset. (This does not have to be formal, but it has to be clear in PIT members' heads.)

3. Keep the membership is as small as possible, but make sure it represents every associate whose "dog is in the fight." Knowing that you'll be asked to join the team when your work is involved is a critical element of trust and empowerment. "On-demand" contacts are helpful.

4. Give clinical PITs resources, including medical records experts, historic data on relevant cases, Medline and article access, and consultants and field trips to excellent-performance HCOs if needed.

5. Set a timetable that expects progress at every meeting, and formal reports at least quarterly. This usually means a support crew working on fact-finding and details.

6. Make sure proposed clinical protocols are pilot-tested. The PIT must find and eliminate bugs; patients are endangered if it does not.

WHAT IS EXCELLENT CARE?

Excellent care is care that correctly identifies and fully meets each patient's healthcare needs. It fulfills the Institute of Medicine (IOM) goals of safe, effective, patient-centered, timely, efficient, and equitable care. Here are some other characteristics of excellent care:

- Excellent care implements evidence-based medicine.
- Excellent care is objectively evaluated. Each IOM goal can be measured and benchmarked. Each clinical unit receives frequent reports. The HCO's strategic scorecard reports HCO achievement on major aggregates.
- Excellent care is financially rewarding. Length of stay and cost per case drop. Improved patient satisfaction attracts market share. Malpractice is avoided and settlement costs are controlled. The HCO and its affiliated physicians benefit in real dollars.

Most HCOs fall short of excellence. Quality, utilization, and patient satisfaction vary substantially between communities, HCOs, and physician specialties.

Community health is a broader definition of excellent care. Excellent individual care is expanded to include unmet community needs and disease prevention. The broader definition must be explicitly adopted as part of the mission and is discussed in Chapter 9.

HOW IS EXCELLENT CARE ACHIEVED?

Excellent HCOs achieve excellent care by:

1. ensuring accurate diagnosis,
2. using standardized processes or protocols, and
3. organizing care teams into service lines treating similar patients.

Exhibit 5.1 describes five functions each service line must perform. Although the details differ, the approach to these functions is standardized across the HCO. A specific treatment, such as an intravenous line, should follow the best practice and be the same in all service lines. A unique intervention, like a cancer therapy treatment, should meet HCO-wide standards. Similarly, although the content for credentialing caregivers differs by specialty and profession, the process should be standard. The result is that high-performing service lines are supported by a shared support structure described in this chapter and chapters 6, 7, and 8.

HOW DOES THE HCO ENSURE ACCURATE DIAGNOSIS?

Accurate diagnosis drives excellent care. The process of diagnosis—identifying and monitoring the patient's condition through symptoms, signs, and diagnostic tests—is ongoing and critical.

Exhibit 5.1 Functions of Service Lines

Function	What the Service Line Does
Ensure accurate diagnosis	Selects effective caregivers and monitors their effectiveness
	Provides training to maintain and improve clinical skills
	Supports responsive listening to patients' needs
	Provides diagnostic clinical support services
Ensure safe, effective, patient-centered, timely, efficient, and equitable care	Updates and maintains protocols
	Trains caregivers in protocol use
	Ensures patient safety and minimizes risks
	Provides informed consent
	Maintains logistic support
	Keeps a record of care
	Coordinates care
Individualize patient care planning and treatment	Provides specialist consultation
	Provides nursing care
	Supports communication among caregivers, patient, family, and subsequent caregivers
Improve community health	Measures community health with a set of indicatorsand benchmarks
	Catalyzes community interest
	Collaborates with other organizations
	Promotes effectiveness
	De-markets unnecessary care
Improve clinical performance	Supports measurement and benchmarking
	Supports PITs
	Uses protocols, training, and incentives to implement improved methods

Accurate diagnosis requires professionals with appropriate skills and a support system that allows them to exercise those skills. An excellent HCO:

1. Provides effective logistics that deliver the information, personnel, supplies, equipment, and facilities for diagnosis. These functions are described in chapters 7 and 8 and chapters 10 through 12.
2. Provides ongoing training that allows professionals to implement the current frontier of science.
3. Ensures competency through credentialing. This assurance—"I can rely on all my teammates"—is a critical component for all associates and for customers, whose rights are clearly established in the law.
4. Ensures competency through training. The HCO's culture must encourage continuous learning and self-improvement. Managers and leaders must be quick to implement new and revised protocols, develop training and development programs for professional and support personnel, and evaluate educational OFIs to tailor training and development plans to each individual.

WHAT ARE THE ADVANTAGES OF PROTOCOLS?

Clinical protocols are consensus statements on the right act in a given set of circumstances. They are formalized, often scientific, responses to specific patient stimuli. They come in two forms:

Functional protocols determine how functional elements of care are carried out. They cover tasks of care accomplished by individuals (such as giving an injection or taking a chest x-ray) and sets of activities for team procedures (such as surgical operations, rehabilitation programs, or multistep diagnostic activities). They are usually written but are often carried out from memory.

Patient management protocols (also called *pathways, guidelines,* or simply *protocols*) define the normal steps or processes in the care of a clinically related group of patients at a specific institution. Patient management protocols are organized around episodes of patient care and are classified by symptom, disease, or condition (such as chest pain, pneumonia, or pregnancy). They specify the functional components of care, outcomes quality goals, and, by implication, the cost.

Protocols are essential to 21st century care:

1. They make coordinated teamwork possible and are necessary to allow the sophisticated 24/7 integration in today's intensive care.
2. They are particularly strong protecting against omission—the forgotten or overlooked step that can create complications, cost, and unsatisfactory outcomes.
3. They provide a foundation for soliciting and implementing the patient's choices in disease management.
4. They provide the basis for assessing or monitoring clinical performance.
5. They reduce length of stay and cost per case.
6. They reduce malpractice errors and provide a more solid defense.
7. They have become a convenient platform for contracts with patients and insurers.

WHAT DOES THE IPOC CONTRIBUTE?

Patient management protocols require continuous adaptation to the patient's evolving condition. The attending physician is obligated to monitor the patient's progress and to modify the protocol to fit the patient's needs. Most patients will require some modification; some patients will require major modification. The interdisciplinary plan of care (IPOC) allows physicians, nurses, and other caregivers to modify the patient's care and maintain a record of changes and additions to the protocol. Goals are developed with the patient for the episode of care, as well as across the trajectory of the illness or condition. The IPOC considers psychosocial and spiritual support, educational needs, cultural and linguistic needs, and community resources and post-discharge planning. A critical aspect of IPOC development is listening to the patient, being vigilant to subtle changes in the patient's condition, and communicating with the attending physician and other caregivers about the patient's progress on plan-of-care goals.

A good IPOC will address all of the following elements:

1. *Assessment*—comprehensive review of the patient's diagnosis, disabilities, and needs, and identification of any unique risks.
2. *Treatment goals*—statement of clinical goals, such as "minimize exacerbation of congestive heart failure," and functional goals, such as "restore ability to dress and feed self."
3. *Component activities*—a list, often selected from relevant care guidelines and functional protocols, of procedures desired for the patient.
4. *Recording*—a formal routine for recording what was done and reporting it to others caring for the patient.
5. *Measures of progress and a schedule for improvement*—where possible, measures of improvement should be used and should parallel the goals developed in the assessment.
6. *Danger signals and counter-indications*—specific events indicating a need to reconsider the plan.

The IPOC forms the basis for coordinating therapeutic services. Unnecessary or ineffective treatment is discouraged. When necessary, the institutional ethics committee is consulted to assist in reaching consensus. In extremely complex cases, it expands into an individual care plan that is often monitored in a formal team process.

HOW ARE PROTOCOLS KEPT EXCELLENT?

Both functional and patient management protocols must be kept current with scientific advances. They are interconnected; a change in one often triggers needs for changes in others.

Functional Protocols

Functional protocols are often the domain of one clinical specialty. The specialty's professional literature instigates and supports revisions. HCO review processes must be more extensive. When an OFI arises involving a functional protocol, a PIT or protocol review team:

1. checks for interactions with other caregivers,
2. uses the relevant patient management protocols to establish the appropriate indications for the function, and
3. pilot-tests any changes to make sure they fit into other care activities.

Good functional protocols have the following components:

1. *Authorization*—statement of who may order the procedure
2. *Indication*—statement clarifying clinical conditions that support the appropriate use of the protocol
3. *Counter-indications*—conditions where the procedure must be modified, replaced, or avoided
4. *Required supplies, equipment, and conditions*—all special requirements and the sources that meet them

5. *Actions*—clear, step-by-step statements of what must be done
6. *Recording*—instructions for recording the procedure and observation of the patient's reaction
7. *Follow-up*—subsequent actions, including checks on the patient's response, measures of effectiveness, indications for repeating the procedure, and disposal or clean-up of supplies

Many functional protocols are linked in sets; pre-operative care and rehabilitation activities are good examples.

An important source of improvement is eliminating unnecessary or inappropriate procedures by making the indications or authorizations more restrictive. For example, elaborate diagnostic tests and expensive drugs can require failure of simpler approaches. Some very expensive procedures can require prior approval or a formal second opinion. The activities themselves can be modified to be safer or less expensive. Changes in equipment and supplies often trigger adjustments. For example, medication administration protocols have changed steadily. The new systems have better controls for reminder alerts to guard against prescribing the wrong drug, administering the wrong dose, or recording the dose incorrectly. The result is lower cost and higher quality.

Patient Management Protocols

Patient management protocols are owned by service lines. They are usually based on publicly available sources such as the National Guideline Clearinghouse (NGC), www.guideline.gov/. As of 2009, the NGC has nearly 2,100 guidelines covering most common diseases and conditions and a number of prevention activities. The Clearinghouse supports several features to aid implementation (www.guideline.gov/about/about.aspx):

1. Structured abstracts (summaries) about each guideline and its development

2. Links to full-text guidelines, where available, and/or ordering information for print copies
3. Palm-based personal digital assistant downloads of the NGC's "Complete Summary" for all guidelines represented in the database
4. A Guideline Comparison utility for a side-by-side comparison of attributes of two or more guidelines
5. Unique guideline comparisons called Guideline Syntheses covering similar topics, highlighting areas of similarity and difference, with international comparisons
6. An electronic forum—NGC-L—for exchanging information on clinical practice guidelines and their development, implementation, and use
7. An annotated bibliography database on guideline development methodology, structure, evaluation, and implementation
8. An Expert Commentary feature

Individual institutions develop protocols by reviewing and revising published guidelines and having a cross-functional PIT explore all the ramifications of the protocol in advance, including trials as necessary. The development process opens the debatable issues and encourages discussion and consensus. It allows the caregivers time to learn new approaches. It checks the proposed guidelines against current practice and pilot-tests to identify areas where new supplies, tools, or training will be required.

HOW ARE PROTOCOLS IMPLEMENTED?

Implementation requires a coordinated effort. The logistic support services—knowledge, human resources, and environment-of-care management—are usually involved. New procedures require new records, new training, and new supplies and equipment. Senior management's role emphasizes effective relationships and coordination. It is their job to see that all these units respond effectively to service line needs. They work through the Performance Improvement Council (PIC) and through their individual assignments to identify, resolve, and remove obstacles.

Functional protocols are implemented by nursing and other clinical support services. Training, coaching, and follow-up assessment are used to ensure compliance. Collaboration with service lines is often necessary.

For patient management protocols, there should be broad consensus within the service line, but uniform compliance is not essential and may not be appropriate. The consensus is built by the PIT. The PIT must find the solution that best fulfills IOM goals, recognizing that trade-offs are inevitable. There must be agreement that the final proposal meets minimum standards—that is superior to the alternative of not offering the service and referring the patient. Most patient management protocols are now linked to specific outcomes and process quality and efficiency measures. The goals are set for these measures. Caregivers are encouraged to integrate the protocol and the IPOC to achieve these goals. Approaching implementation through the quality goals allows individual physicians to use the IPOC to see for themselves whether their innovations improve results.

Success requires both a cultural (Chapter 2) and an operational (Chapter 3) foundation. The cultural foundation is an expansion of the values of respect and compassion, and of the values shared by most clinical professions, as shown in Exhibit 5.2. The HCO advertises its commitment to the values. Recruitment emphasizes the philosophy of the organization so that it attracts doctors and employees who are congenial to its orientation. Decisions of PITs and PICs and daily activities consistently reinforce these values. An ethics committee is available to advise on complex applications.

Exhibit 5.2 Core Values of High-Performing HCOs

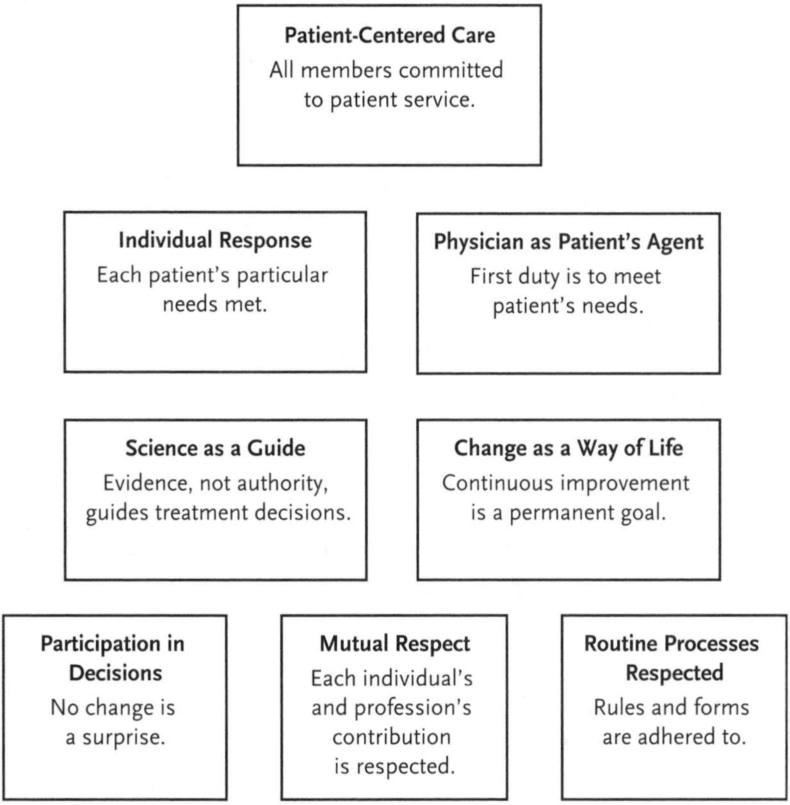

Patient-Centered Care
All members committed
to patient service.

Individual Response
Each patient's particular
needs met.

Physician as Patient's Agent
First duty is to meet
patient's needs.

Science as a Guide
Evidence, not authority,
guides treatment decisions.

Change as a Way of Life
Continuous improvement
is a permanent goal.

**Participation in
Decisions**
No change is
a surprise.

Mutual Respect
Each individual's
and profession's
contribution
is respected.

**Routine Processes
Respected**
Rules and forms
are adhered to.

SHOULD OUR HCO ADOPT A COMMUNITY HEALTH MISSION?

HCOs differ in the extent to which they pursue prevention and health promotion. Those with an "excellence in care" mission focus on services that occur between the caregiver and the individual patient. Those with a "community health" mission incorporate broader efforts to minimize disease and its impact. Chapter 9 addresses the distinction and its implications as well as strategies for improving community health.

HCOs provide prevention and health promotion for four reasons:

1. The moral commitment of all caregiving professionals is to health, clearly including prevention.
2. Prevention opportunities arise from the same scientific knowledge as treatment opportunities. More than 1,300 of the NGC guidelines reference prevention, and the number is increasing.[1]
3. Healthcare professionals are respected authority figures, and their advice is given at times when the patient is receptive. Their support legitimizes preventive behavior.
4. Prevention helps communities that own HCOs. Each episode of illness prevented translates eventually to reductions in cost of care. A healthier community has more workers and lower health insurance costs, making it a better place to build or expand a business.

Prevention and health promotion tools can be used to change behavior on three levels:

- **Primary prevention** activities are those that take place before the disease occurs to eliminate or reduce its occurrence. Immunizations, seat belts, condoms, sewage treatment, and restrictions on alcohol sales are examples.
- **Secondary prevention** reduces the consequences of disease, often by early detection and treatment. Self-examination; routine dental inspections;

---

[1]National Guideline Clearinghouse. 2009. [Online information; retrieved 5/27/09.] www.guideline.gov/search/searchresults.aspx?Type=3&txtSearch=prevention&num=20.

mammographies; colonoscopies; and management of chronic diseases like diabetes, hypertension, and asthma are examples.

- **Tertiary prevention** is the avoidance of complications or sequelae. Early physical therapy for strokes, retraining in activities of daily living, and respite services to help family caregivers are examples. Chronic diseases also present numerous tertiary prevention opportunities.

Functional and patient management protocols should incorporate all categories of prevention and health promotion. For example, functional protocols for injections, surgical interventions, and other treatments prevent hospital-acquired infections and injury to caregivers. Home care visit protocols include inspection for hazards and discussion of patient needs and symptoms with family members. Diabetic and cardiovascular care protocols include selection of the optimal pharmacological treatment and guidance to the patient in lifestyle and nutrition. Prenatal, postnatal, and child care protocols include immunizations; checks for potential developmental disabilities; and education for the mother on child development, nutrition, home safety, and domestic violence.

Ironically, primary and tertiary disease prevention reduces hospital and physician revenues. Well-managed institutions do both anyway; it is part of excellent care and probably essential to avoid bankrupting the major healthcare financing programs. HCOs with a community mission pursue primary and tertiary prevention aggressively. Secondary prevention usually increases hospital and physician revenues. It is also the most scientifically controversial prevention area. Prostate cancer and breast cancer screenings have been strenuously challenged to meet clinical and cost effectiveness criteria. HCOs with a community mission will encourage compliance with the published guidelines, but not beyond them.

HOW IS CLINICAL PERFORMANCE MEASURED AND IMPROVED?

Accountability for clinical operations now requires a complex structure, as shown in Exhibit 5.3. Both service lines and support services actively seek OFIs and implement them through PITs. Most PITs require members from several teams. An OFI for angiography practices would require input from primary care, cardiology and emergency service lines, imaging, anesthesia, nursing, pharmacy, and laboratory (any team whose activities might be affected). Most teams and associates in nursing and clinical support services have dual reporting, through their service lines and their profession. A quality management office serves as a consultative resource. It is essential for the senior management team leaders to coordinate closely—"joined at the hip," as one COO put it.

Exhibit 5.4 shows the operational scorecard template for a service line and its component units. The details will differ, particularly in the demand and quality measures, among service lines. In most applications, a few measures are selected in each dimension for goal-setting. Those that have achieved benchmark or that are not candidates for improvement can be dropped and replaced by others better related to current needs. The dropped measures remain available for analyzing OFIs. When the service line is separately incorporated, it is possible to construct a strategic scorecard for it as well. Strategic scorecards are required for joint ventures.

The epidemiologic planning model constructs demand forecasts from available community information. Outcomes and process quality measures have expanded substantially in recent years. The new measures often contain sophisticated adjustments to remove factors beyond the service's control. They have become practical as electronic record keeping has expanded. These are the main sources of measures:

- The National Quality Measures Clearinghouse, www.qualitymeasures.ahrq.gov/, is the starting point for any discussion of clinical performance measurement.

Exhibit 5.3 Organization of Clinical Services

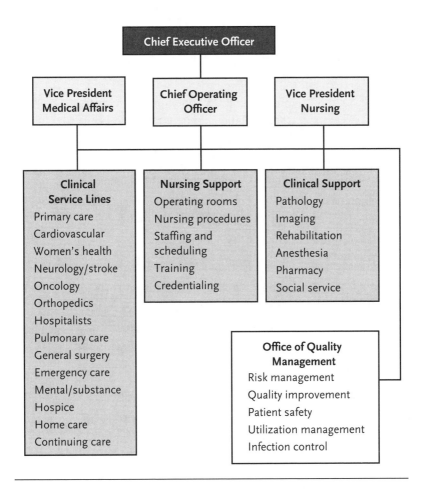

- The Joint Commission National Patient Safety Goals, www.jointcommission.org/PatientSafety/National PatientSafetyGoals/09_hap_npsgs.htm, promote specific improvements in patient safety.
- The Leapfrog Group, www.leapfroggroup.org/, calculates regional outcomes quality, efficiency, and effectiveness scores on a battery of common inpatient diseases.

Exhibit 5.4 Profile of Service Line Operational Scorecard

Dimensions	Examples
Input Measures	
Demand	
Requests for care	Patient arrivals, appointment requests, consultation and referral requests
	Often specified by patient age, service, and location
Market share	Percent of total demand from community
Appropriateness of service	Percent of expected or benchmark demand from epidemiologic planning model
Logistics of service	Hours of availability
Cost/Resources	
Total costs per patient	Labor, supplies, plant, indirect costs for service line
Resource condition	Occupancy and percent of capacity rates, age of equipment, failure rates of equipment
Human Resources	
Supply	Staffing levels, staffing shortfalls, vacancy rates
Training	Average hours of training per associate
Employee satisfaction	Associate loyalty, retention or termination, absenteeism, work loss days from accident or injury
Output Measures	
Output/ Productivity	
Patients treated	Discharge counts by specified group
Cost per case	Total costs/discharges by specified group
Cost per treatment	Costs for specific activity such as surgical operations or examinations/patients receiving

Exhibit 5.4 *Continued*

Dimensions	Examples
Output Measures	
Quality	
Clinical outcomes	Outcomes assess patient condition at discharge
Procedural quality	Procedural measures assess completion of specific tasks or events
Structural quality	Structural measures assess availability and adequacy of service, particularly staffing and facility safety
Customer Satisfaction	
Patient satisfaction	Post-discharge surveys, counts of "Caught in the Act," complaints, service recovery, and unexpected incidents
Referring physician satisfaction	Surveys, rounding, complaints
Other customer satisfaction	Community surveys, boundary-spanning activities
Access	Delays for service, unfilled demand

- The National Quality Forum, www.qualityforum.org, endorses 34 practices that should be universally used in clinical settings to reduce the risk of harm to patients. Structural measures of quality—basically counts of availability of appropriate resources—are now rarely useful for quality assessment.
- The Agency for Healthcare Research and Quality, www.ahrq.gov/qual/hospsurvey09/hosp09summ.htm, has a "Hospital Survey of Patient Safety Culture," which assesses associates' perceptions of the clinical culture.

WHERE ARE THE STUMBLING BLOCKS?

Reaching clinical excellence is the central challenge for any HCO management. Here are several recurring issues and how successful HCOs approach them:

1. **Credentialing and Ensuring Continued Competence**
   The issue is how to deal with the occasional professional who is not making the grade. The best response is careful monitoring of ongoing performance coupled with personal interviews, counseling, and a step-wise program of correction. Failure to act on early signals has serious consequences. Although expensive and difficult for the individuals involved, direct supervision can protect patients from serious harm, and the HCO from massive costs. Only after these efforts have failed is it necessary to withdraw approval. By that time, the case is usually ironclad.

2. **Minimizing and Responding to Unanticipated Clinical Events**   Protocols, credentialing, and continuous improvement substantially reduce the chance of error, but unanticipated clinical events still occur. The method for dealing with these events is now clearly established and documented. It calls for rigorous application of the following rules:

   a. Every unanticipated clinical event with negative consequences for the patient should be reported by the caregiving team involved.

   b. Minor events become candidates for service recovery (Chapter 11) and OFIs for continuous improvement.

   c. Major events are thoroughly and objectively reviewed. The HCO reaches a decision about liability. If it is liable, it offers an appropriate, immediate financial settlement. If it is not liable, it offers its sympathy and appropriate non-financial support. If its offers are not acceptable to patients or survivors, the HCO allows the matter to proceed to mediation or trial.

d. The record of major events is systematically studied for OFIs.

Under this approach, there is no malpractice crisis. The HCO should go to court rarely, and only when it expects to win. The cost of settlement is much less than the cost of defense, and the OFIs revealed steadily reduce the incidence of events.[2]

3. **Resolving Interprofessional Rivalries**   As noted, protocols frequently allow less skilled personnel to provide care under supervision by more skilled staff, but these substitutions create potential income losses for the original providers. Well-managed organizations must be sensitive to these concerns, but they must move steadily toward using the lowest-cost provider that is safe and effective. The guides under the "What Are Some Good Responses to Common Issues?" section in Chapter 2 must be applied. The epidemiologic planning model allows orderly change in supply. The participants must leave the debate thinking that they were fairly treated. Stakeholders must not be allowed to use economic power to stymie progress for all.

4. **Implementing the Electronic Record**   The electronic medical record (EMR) facilitates excellent care; it is not essential. Protocols and IPOCs are proven to contribute with paper and transitional records. The return on investment from the EMR depends heavily on the effectiveness of service lines and the extra gains in patient care. Most of the current high performing HCOs built the culture and operational infrastructure first, and moved later to automate the supporting record.

---

[2]Boothman, R. C., A. C. Blackwell, D. A. Campbell, Jr., E. Commiskey, and S. Anderson. 2009. "A Better Approach to Medical Malpractice Claims? The University of Michigan Experience." *Journal of Health and Life Sciences Law* 2 (2): 125–159.

5. **Small HCOs**   Excellent care requires an array of clinical support services, specialist consultation, and referrals. A large team of qualified specialists is obviously an asset, but rural communities cannot support more than a few people. Formal affiliations with larger centers are superior to individual patient referrals, assuming the larger center can document excellent care. Affiliation establishes a commitment to practical service; allows sharing of expensive resources, such as magnetic resonance imagers; supports measured performance and annual goal-setting; and can include educational services and advice on protocols. Telemedicine and referral linkages are making remote consultation more practical, extending services to rural areas.

6. **Strategic Support**   High-performing HCOs work strategically with markets and money. Each service is sized according to its epidemiologic needs. Market share is enhanced because patients are delighted. New equipment is available because funds were on hand to buy it. Credentialing standards can be upheld because the organization pursues recruitment and individual development aggressively. The underlying reason that it can afford to do this is that care that meets IOM goals is inherently less costly than care that falls short.

SUGGESTED READINGS

Black, J., with D. Miller. 2008. *The Toyota Way to Healthcare Excellence: Increase Efficiency and Improve Quality with Lean.* Chicago: Health Administration Press.

Carroll, R. (ed.). 2010. *Risk Management Handbook for Health Care Organizations,* 5th Edition. San Francisco: Jossey-Bass.

The Joint Commission. *Accreditation Standards* (published annually). Oakbrook Terrace, IL: The Joint Commission.

Kelly, D. L. 2006. *Applying Quality Management in Healthcare: A Systems Approach,* 2nd ed. Chicago: Health Administration Press.

Nelson, E. C., P. B. Batalden, and M. M. Godfrey (eds.). 2007. *Quality by Design: A Clinical Microsystems Approach.* San Francisco: Jossey-Bass.

Chapter 6   In a Few Words . . .

The excellent HCO is the major vehicle for negotiating physicians' contribution to a community's healthcare. The collaboration determines the supply of physicians, thus indirectly physician income and health insurance costs. The physician organization, now built around service lines:

1. implements systems for improving the quality and efficiency of care;
2. approves the credentials and monitors the performance of individual physicians;
3. assists in planning the number and kinds of doctors;
4. conducts continuing education for its members and other caregivers;
5. provides a network of communication between physicians, other associates, and the governing board;
6. participates in designing compensation and risk-sharing arrangements.
7. monitors and improves its own effectiveness as an organization.

The performance of physicians is measured directly from patient care; the performance of the physician organization is measured primarily by its effectiveness in recruiting and retaining members. The HCO's goal is to offer each physician a place to practice excellent medicine, with similarly committed colleagues and reliable organizational support.

The Physician Organization

care, so that it supports specialist income. (If their mission is community health, they work on transferring patients back to primary care promptly and avoiding unnecessary specialist care.)

4. They make protocols work. Protocols are carefully planned and tested, kept up to date, and flexibly applied. Other caregivers are carefully trained. Logistics are transparent—each doctor has what she needs, when she needs it, before she asks.

5. They work to maximize physician net income. They eliminate burdensome processes, provide knowledgeable non-physician caregivers, run practices, engage in joint ventures, negotiate solid insurance contracts, and minimize malpractice risk, so that income opportunities remain competitive.

What to Do Next?

Medical practice by its very nature raises some recurring problems.

Your coach says, "Excellent HCOs have established processes to deal with the 'frequently asked questions' in physician-HCO relationships." You want to be able to answer these common questions with these answers:

1. *"I need a competent clinical consultant."*
   "You can trust your colleagues here because we credential carefully and monitor clinical performance. We have an arrangement with (prominent local referral center) to facilitate super-specialist referrals and consultations if you want to use it."

2. *"I need reliable nurse, lab, imaging, anesthesia, etc."*
   "We pursue continuous improvement and 'state of the art' excellence in all clinical support services.

Each service and unit has goals in quality, patient satisfaction, and physician satisfaction. We're proud that many are near national benchmark. We want to hear about any serious issue that arises."

3. *"I need more time."*

"Don't we all! But we have several ways to save you time: electronic medical records, well-trained support personnel, convenient parking, nearby offices, office management, and training for your personnel. If you let us, we can fix it so that you spend almost all of every day actually caring for patients."

4. *"I need more net income."*

"Our services to save you time can also save you money. And we're open to any reasonable financial arrangement. We can talk about employment, joint ventures, joint insurance contracts, or straight fee-for-service. If it's legal, and makes business sense, we're willing to try it."

5. *"I had an unexpected clinical event."*

"Sorry to hear that, but these things happen, and we're prepared for it. We need the details, and we'll do an investigation. Our first goal is prevention. We've reduced events that lead to HCO or physician liability."

The 20th century saw a revolution in medical practice. Medical care became a team event rather than a one-to-one relationship. Physicians became team leaders coordinating the work of a dozen or more caregivers. With the growth of scientific medicine and protocols, "evidence" replaced "judgment" as the criterion for quality.[1] The revolution has been incompletely and unevenly

[1] Evidence-Based Working Group. 1992. "Evidence-Based Medicine. A New Approach to Teaching the Practice of Medicine." *JAMA* 268 (17): 2420–25.

deployed to actual patients, and it has created substantial turmoil for practicing physicians. In the early 21st century, about 20 percent of doctors were unhappy with their profession. Satisfaction varies substantially by geographic location.

The excellent HCO advances the revolution and improves physician satisfaction. The purpose of its physician organization is:

to recruit and retain physicians necessary to provide excellent care to the community.

This purpose uses the HCO as a framework for a negotiated relationship between the community stakeholders and the physicians. The HCO offers:

- access without charge to facilities, equipment, and trained personnel essential to the physician's practice;
- empowerment to participate in ongoing change;
- a culture of respect, compassion, and commitment to excellence; and
- direct and indirect financial support.

In return, the HCO asks the physician for:

- commitment to its mission;
- compliance with its rules and procedures; and
- maintenance of professional competence.

Like all close relationships, this one is potentially stressful. The framework of the physician organization must be robust enough to withstand the stresses that arise and respond to them in a constructive manner. In excellent HCOs, the physician organization fulfills the six major functions shown in Exhibit 6.1.

Exhibit 6.1 Functions of the Physician Organization

Function	Contribution	Examples
Achieve excellent care	Provide high quality, cost-effective health care	Continuous improvement of care through clinical protocols, case management, and prevention
Credential and privilege physicians and related professionals	Ensure continued effectiveness and reliability of all clinical teams	Recruitment and selection of new members, renewal of privileges
Plan and implement physician recruitment	Ensure an adequate supply of well-trained physicians	Physician-needs planning, recruitment
Provide clinical education for physicians and other professionals	Ensure a well-trained body of caregivers	Case reviews, protocol development, scientific programs, and graduate medical education
Negotiate collective compensation	Allow customer access to a full range of healthcare financing opportunities	Negotiation and implementation of risk-sharing contracts with payers and intermediaries
Collaborate on continuous improvement	Bring clinical viewpoint to all activities of the organization	Governing board, strategic planning, budgeting participation

WHAT DOES THE 21ST CENTURY PHYSICIAN CONTRIBUTE?

The Accreditation Council for Graduate Medical Education has identified six competencies of physicians generally:[2]

1. **Patient care** that is compassionate, appropriate, and effective for the treatment of health problems and the promotion of health

2. **Medical knowledge** about established and evolving biomedical, clinical, and cognate (e.g., epidemiological and social-behavioral) sciences and the application of this knowledge to patient care

3. **Practice-based learning and improvement** that involves investigation and evaluation of their own patient care, appraisal and assimilation of scientific evidence, and improvements in patient care

4. **Interpersonal and communication skills** that result in effective information exchange and teaming with patients, their families, and other health professionals

5. **Professionalism**, as manifested through a commitment to carrying out professional responsibilities, adherence to ethical principles, and sensitivity to a diverse patient population

6. **Systems-based practice**, as manifested by actions that demonstrate an awareness of and responsiveness to the larger context and system of healthcare and the ability to effectively call on system resources to provide care that is of optimal value

The first three—patient care, medical knowledge, and improvement through practice—are part of the long history of professional

---

[2]Accreditation Council for Graduate Medical Education. 2009. [Online information; retrieved 7/14/09.] www.acgme.org/outcome/comp/compMin.asp.

medicine. Most medical specialties now provide programs of various kinds and test for continued competence at regular intervals. By requiring continued certification and by selecting and installing current protocols, the HCO ensures maintenance of these competencies. These skills support the reliability of the medical staff. Any physician's clinical opinion, expressed in an interdisciplinary plan of care (IPOC), on a protocol review committee, or in a consultation or referral can be trusted as professionally competent.

The last three—interpersonal and communications skills, professionalism, and systems-based practice—are important for all physicians, and they will be increasingly important in the 21st century. The HCO strengthens these and relies on them to build an effective system.

HOW DOES THE PHYSICIAN ORGANIZATION SUPPORT EXCELLENT CARE?

Service-line based excellence builds upon the similarity of patient needs and the specialized skills of caregivers. It is summarized in the central structure of Exhibit 6.2. It applies not simply to acute care specialties but to all healthcare, from primary offices to post acute care. Every service line requires the supporting services shown in the two sidebars: clinical support for continuing diagnosis, specialized treatments, and implementation of the IPOC and operational support, including marketing and strategic positioning.

There are currently three approaches to filling the sidebar needs: (1) free-standing cottage industry solutions purchase or arrange the services from vendors in strategic partnerships or on an "as needed" basis; (2) national specialty firms, such as DaVita in dialysis and Beverly Enterprises in nursing homes, provide the needs with national organizations focused on single service lines; and (3) integrated HCOs provide the services to a broad range of service lines and fulfill comprehensive health needs.

Exhibit 6.2 Service Line Excellence and Support Needs

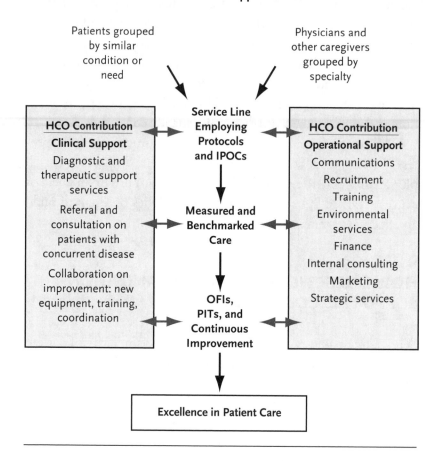

Most community hospitals and healthcare systems are committed to the third approach. There are a lot of theoretical reasons that it should prevail, but it will actually prevail only if it is superior in the marketplace. That means:

1. It is better at meeting patient needs:

   • Each service line operates at or near benchmark on quality, patient satisfaction, and cost.

- Clinical and operational support services are provided at a level superior to what can be offered by independent vendors.
- The "single source" concept is successfully promoted to patients.

2. It is better at satisfying caregiver needs:

- Each caregiver associate feels empowered and supported by the central organization.
- The values and culture of the organization make it an attractive place to practice.
- Earning opportunities are competitive. The HCO's brand and promotion add economic value for the caregiver.

High-performing HCOs are winning the competitive battle. Their physician organizations contribute to these goals by maintaining the performance of individual physicians, providing empowered cultures and continuous improvement infrastructures, and deliberately protecting physician income while meeting community-based needs. Excellence in clinical support services, logistic services, and strategic services is also necessary, as Exhibit 6.2 shows.

WHAT IS THE RIGHT WAY TO CREDENTIAL PHYSICIANS?

Credentialing is the guarantee of competence the HCO provides for its patient and customer stakeholders, and also for its associate stakeholders. The process used for physicians is the oldest and most formalized. It remains occasionally contentious, but in excellent HCOs it is simply expected and routine. The core action, monitoring actual behavior, is centered at the level of the teams within the service lines or clinical support services. Here is how physician credentialing works in excellent HCOs:

1. Applications are accepted only for vacancies generated by the planning process (see below).
2. Every applicant is thoroughly screened. The appropriate specialty selects the best qualified applicants, based on the screening information.
3. Privileges are precisely specified in terms of clinical procedures or duties, and are limited to two years.
4. Performance is monitored and measured.
5. Early warning and intervention is used whenever questions arise.
6. There is an emergency intervention system in the bylaws that ensures control of unexpected and unacceptable behavior.
7. Physicians who do not respond to intervention are suspended or their credentials are not renewed. The review process is clearly spelled out in medical staff bylaws. The actions are supported by a clear record of cases and statistics on performance.
8. There is a formal appeals process in the bylaws. Cases going to appeal are infrequent, and the appellant must overcome substantial documentation of cause.

Steps 1 through 5 are built into the HCO's ongoing routine and culture. They set the tone—professional practice is expected at all times, and occasional weaknesses are treated as learning opportunities. They require employed physician leadership and substantial technical support from the HCO. Step 4 requires a full implementation of performance measures in each service line (Exhibit 5.4) and clinical support service (Exhibits 7.5 and 8.4). Step 5 requires that physician leadership be fully trained in identifying and pursing early warning signals. A program for recovery from substance abuse is a valuable component. The significant financial investment involved in building this system is recovered from improved patient care, reduced incidence of steps 6 though 8, and reduced malpractice costs.

WHY SHOULD THE HCO PLAN PHYSICIAN SUPPLY?

The HCO lacks the authority to deny a physician the right to open or close a practice. But it can deny access to the hospital and recruit for caregivers based on community need. An excellent HCO will rigorously analyze community needs, opportunities, and strategies to ensure the right number of physicians. In doing so, it protects its physicians from competition and offers that protection as part of its privileging contract. It avoids anti-trust implications by keeping final control of the plan securely in the hands of the governing board.

A shortage of physicians has obvious implications: waiting lines, insufficient service, omitted care, and patients seeking care in other areas. It also has some not-so-obvious implications: overworked and stressed caregivers, loss of appropriate community income, higher complication of presenting patients, and higher risk of unfavorable care events. An oversupply of physicians has serious implications as well: reduced individual incomes, a tendency toward unnecessary care, and insufficient practice to maintain technical skills. Both oversupply and undersupply can lead to excess health insurance costs. The HCO's plans strive for balance: every caregiver has enough activity to maintain skills and the income they desire, and all appropriate patient needs are locally met in a timely fashion.

HOW DOES THE HCO PLAN PHYSICIAN SUPPLY?

The healthcare institution must make capital investments to support the physician supply. The investment decisions are part of the strategic or long-range plan of the institution discussed in Chapter 15. Decisions are made first on the question of scope of service—"Should we have a cardiovascular surgery program?"—and second on the actual facilities and number of physicians required. As illustrated in Exhibit 6.3, the physician recruitment plan is an extension of these decisions.

The general epidemiologic planning model discussed in Chapter 3 is applied to each specialty of the physician organization. The work intentions of currently privileged practitioners—anticipated retirements, reduced or increased workloads—are obtained by survey. The difference between the need estimated by the epidemiologic planning model and the supply found by the survey is the anticipated unmet need or surplus.

The process is not perfect. While the incidence of disease is relatively predictable, procedures to treat a disease and what specialty uses them change unpredictably. New technology and improved protocols change the kind of response and the specialty required. (For example, the use of angioplasty, stents, and coronary artery surgery is a dynamic arena, affecting the numbers of cardiovascular surgeons and invasive cardiologists.) Patient acceptance of alternative sources of care is not uniform (the acceptance of midwives is an example). The modeling results must be carefully studied in the light of market conditions.

Good practice calls for carefully analyzing the present situation and exploring a range of possible revisions and their consequences. A forecast of incidence based on local history is usually obtained through the cross-functional teams and the specialties involved. It supplements the need estimate generated by the epidemiologic planning model. Published scientific opinion should be reviewed. Several guidelines—such as values for staff model HMOs, benchmark values for similar-sized cities, and adjustment for anticipated insurance trends—should be considered to evaluate current levels and show the alternative implications for physician supply.

Most HCOs will find a shortage for various primary care specialties. Some HCOs find surpluses in interventional specialties.

Exhibit 6.3 Cardiac Surgery as an Example of Combined Strategic, Service, and Physician Planning

Planning Step	Example	Result
Environmental assessment; mission and vision	Will service population support advanced inpatient referral services?	Adequate demand for referral services in general
Strategic plans and long-range financial plans	What are priority health needs? Which can be met at a competitive price, and which can be served by others?	Cardiovascular surgery is one of several services under consideration
Service line plans and recruitment plans	Forecasts for number of procedures, professional personnel, other personnel, facilities and equipment	Recruitment of cardiovascular surgeon(s) and team(s)
Implementation and goal-setting	Review of actual volumes, outcomes, costs	Continuation, expansion, or contraction of cardiovascular program

The analysis should be used to stimulate discussion among physicians and the governing board. Widespread understanding of the opportunities will improve individual decision making. Discussion may prompt early retirements, relocations, or recruitment opportunities.

The governing board is obligated to address indications of undersupply and severe oversupply. In general, high-cost, low-volume specialties should be carefully justified before the institution commits capital and personnel. A plan to provide a specific referral specialty service affirms that sufficient local demand will exist to maintain the quality and to justify the cost. Oversupplies must be carefully managed. Solutions may require several years to implement, but the board has an obligation to equitable and effective uses of community resources.

HOW DOES AN HCO RECRUIT PHYSICIANS?

Most communities must recruit physicians. Population growth, aging, and retirements of the current staff create vacancies that must be filled. Good physicians have their choice of practice locations, and they are actively recruited even in times of relative surplus. A strategy emphasizing physician extenders is appropriate. A sound approach will promote discussion of the issue among all affected groups, leading to recommendations from the physician organization and final acceptance by the governing board.

A recruitment offer frequently includes arrangements for office facilities and services, income guarantees, health insurance participation contracts, malpractice coverage, membership in a medical partnership or group, and introductions to referring physicians or available specialists. A substantial capital resource is necessary. At the same time, physicians want to work where their colleagues are capable and friendly. Complex offers require early assurance that medical credentials are acceptable, and selecting the right candidate involves assessment of clinical skills. Recruitment is commonly a collaborative activity with existing physician groups. The HCO's support contributes to success.

WHAT TRAINING SHOULD AN HCO OFFER ITS MEDICAL STAFF?

Continuing clinical education is now largely provided by journals and professional associations, but the HCO's review of clinical protocols is an important learning exercise for all practitioners. The HCO must train its current and future leaders in the three new competencies of practice: interpersonal and communications skill, commitment to ethical principles, and systems-based practice. The first two of these are often taught and reinforced principally by example and coaching. The HCO's commitment to these competencies should be clearly and uniformly expressed, and new staff leaders should understand both the content and the activity. Systems-based practice can be taught with leadership training and work process analysis, such as Six Sigma or Lean. Physician leadership education is increasingly driven by the continuous improvement process. Analysis of past performance, benchmarking, the design of new processes, and the preparation of protocols are educational activities in themselves, affecting the quality improvement, credentialing, planning, and educational functions simultaneously.

HOW DOES THE HCO IMPACT PHYSICIAN COMPENSATION?

The HCO's goal in all compensation is a "fair" income, one that is equivalent to what would be earned in a similar effort elsewhere. The concept is clear and intuitively acceptable to most people, but it is difficult to measure, because a great many variables are involved in "equivalent," "similar effort," and "elsewhere." As of 2010, most physicians earn most of their income from modified versions of fee-for-service payment, but they are also compensated directly by the HCO. They also purchase services from the HCO. Five types of contracts underlie the arrangements:

1. *Salary,* for patient care or for managerial activity
2. Contracts providing *office management*
3. *Sale of existing practices,* either to the HCO or by the organization to new physicians
4. *Collective contracts with insurance intermediaries,* offering physicians increased access to insured populations
5. *Joint investment ventures,* offering physicians the opportunity to make an equity investment with the anticipation of return and a salable asset

Each of these mechanisms establishes a different patient-care incentive for the physician, and no incentive perfectly matches all patients' needs. The evidence of improved effectiveness resulting from the incentives is mixed, but it is likely that all five of these devices will become more common. The incentives enhance or detract from other organizational mechanisms, such as the overall culture, the effectiveness of protocol support, and the measurement of critical performance variables.

Tax, inurement, and fraud issues must be avoided by careful design in all of these approaches. Collective contracts and joint investments make the HCO and its physicians economic partners in pursuit of incentive payments. Many states have laws regulating physician incentive compensation. Excellent HCOs always obtain legal counsel for financial contracts with physicians.

WHAT BUILDS MEDICAL STAFF LOYALTY?

In a national report on physician perspectives on U.S. hospitals, three of the top five physician priorities regarding the physician-hospital relationship dealt with how well the HCO's senior leaders communicate, respond, and collaborate with physicians to meet their practice needs.[3] Engaged physicians demonstrate the following traits:

- *Investment*—physicians have an emotional relationship with the hospital, share in its mission and values, and have a sense of pride in their association with the organization.
- *Involvement*—physicians take an active role in improving hospital performance and join with the HCO in providing excellent care.
- *Advocacy*—physicians demonstrate behaviors that build the brand of the HCO by recommending the HCO to patients, physician colleagues, and the community at large.[4]

In order to engage physicians, HCO leaders must listen attentively to their needs and concerns, involve them in decision making, make an effort to understand the language of medicine and what their physicians contribute to excellent patient care, and show them that they value them. Organizations with high levels of physician engagement:

- increase referrals from engaged physicians;
- receive higher net earnings per admission;
- reduce physician recruiting costs; and
- sustain significant growth and profitability.[5]

---

[3]Press Ganey Associates, Inc. 2008. *Hospital Check-Up Report—Physician Perspectives on American Hospitals.* South Bend, IN: Press Ganey Associates, Inc.

[4]Paller, D. 2009. "Physician Partnership: Creating Powerful Relationships." Press Ganey Associates, Inc. [Online information; retrieved 7/14/09.] www.pressganey.com/galleries/default-file/Physician_Partnership_Creating_Powerful_Relationships.pdf.

[5]Gallup. 2009. "Physician Engagement." [Online information; retrieved 7/14/09.] www.gallup.com/consulting/healthcare/15385/Physician-Engagement.aspx.

Most important, engaged physicians with higher levels of satisfaction contribute to the overall mission of providing excellent patient care.

The first step is extensive and open communication. Excellent HCOs make multiple systematic efforts to build a communicating culture empowering every member of the medical staff:

1. Physician representatives are included in all major decision discussions, as shown in Exhibit 6.4.
2. Senior managers devote significant time to individual and group contact with physicians.
3. Formal surveys are used to measure physician satisfaction, as with other associates.
4. Physician leaders, like all managers, are trained to listen, respond effectively, and report.
5. Physicians are invited to serve on the governing board.
6. Maintaining the medical staff structure as well as service lines provides multiple avenues for discussion of most issues.
7. Formal mechanisms for conflict resolution are built into the medical staff bylaws but are used as a last resort.

The goal is a structure in which every physician is empowered and is confident that his voice will be heard in decisions affecting their practice. All physicians should be close to someone whom they respect and who can hear their concerns and either resolve them or explain how they can participate in the resolution.

If all staff members are confident of their empowerment, much can be accomplished through informal discussions. In well-run HCOs, non-medical managers make a deliberate effort

Exhibit 6.4 Physician Representation on Decision Processes

Decision Type	Example	Physician Participation
Mission/vision	Visioning exercise	Extensive individual participation
		Seats on review committees
		Governing board membership
Resource allocation	Environment assessment	Governing board membership
	Strategic plans	Participation in annual review
	Services plan	Membership on board planning and finance committees
	Financial plan	
	Facilities plan	Representation on committees and consultation for services directly involved
	Human resources plan	
	Physician recruitment plan	Advice from each specialty unit
		Opportunity for individual comment
	Budgeting	Participation between line units and services particularly involved
	Capital budgeting	Major voice in ranking all clinical equipment purchases
		Participation in general ranking of capital equipment

Continued

Exhibit 6.4 *Continued*

Decision Type	Example	Physician Participation
Clinical care issues	Process design	Participation by service line in all patient management protocol development
		Review of relevant functional protocols
		Participation or consultation in clinical PITs
Organizational	Personnel selection	Credentialing of all physicians
		Participation on executive search committees
	Implementation plans	Participation by service line
	Information plan	Participation in plan and relevant pilot programs
	Conflict resolution	Membership in mediation efforts and appeals panels

to maintain informal communications with the medical staff, even going to their offices to meet them. By visiting physicians in their offices, hospital managers and executives demonstrate their understanding of the value of a physician's time and show a willingness to become acquainted with physicians on a more personal level.

The practice of providing designated positions on the board for the physicians has become almost universal and is an important advantage of community-based HCOs. Physicians nominate their colleagues in many organizations. To satisfy tax exemption rules, physicians are limited to a substantial minority. These few individuals cannot represent the complex needs of all physicians. Like other board members, they are expected to vote for the best interests of the community, rather than for any short-term advantage to themselves or to the physicians in general. They serve the medical staff more by making sure the physicians' opinions are fully understood and fairly heard than by any specific representation.

The communication network does not solve every problem. Conflicts arise between specialties, between clinical support services and attending physicians, between the HCO and specialty groups, and between individual physicians. Painful sacrifices may be involved in settling them. The organization's bylaws should specify the roles of each office and standing committee of the physician organization and the methods by which communication is encouraged and disagreements are resolved. For disagreements that are particularly serious, the negotiation and conflict resolution approaches described in Chapter 2 are applicable.

HOW CAN AN HCO IMPROVE ITS PHYSICIAN ORGANIZATION?

Like any other accountable unit of the organization, the physician organization should have measures of performance and negotiated improvement goals for the coming year. All service lines have operational measures, as indicated in Exhibit 5.4. Incorporated service lines should have strategic scorecards adding financial measures. In either structure, physician satisfaction is explicitly monitored. It is also possible to evaluate the medical staff as a whole, and activities crossing service lines. Exhibit 6.5 suggests some approaches that will identify OFIs for the physician organization and its components. The use of an outside consultant to conduct an objective review is often effective.

Exhibit 6.5 Operational Measures of Physician Organization Performance

Dimension	Applicable Measures
Demand	Difficult to measure except by associate satisfaction
Cost	Cost budgets for assigned functions
Associate satisfaction	Surveys of physician satisfaction
	Meeting attendance
	Incidents causing excessive disruption
Outcomes and efficiency	Cost per physician served can be calculated and compared to similar organizations.
	Review by internal or external consultants
Operations	Review by internal or external consultants
	Items arising from associate satisfaction
Customer satisfaction	Patient quality and satisfaction surveys measure the ultimate customer satisfaction.
	The physicians are internal customers, and they are monitored as "associates," above.
	Other service lines are also internal customers (e.g., primary care is a customer of most specialties). Satisfaction with those relationships can be included in physician surveys.

SUGGESTED READINGS

Cohn, K. H. 2005. *Better Communication for Better Care: Mastering Physician-Administrator Collaboration.* Chicago: Health Administration Press.

Gassiot, C. A., V. L. Searcy, and C. W. Giles. 2007. *The Medical Staff Services Handbook: Fundamentals and Beyond.* Sudbury, MA: Jones and Bartlett.

Hammon, J. L. (ed.). 2000. *Fundamentals of Medical Management: A Guide for the Physician Executive,* 2nd edition. Tampa, FL: American College of Physician Executives.

Warden, J. 2009. *Creating Sustainable Physician-Hospital Strategies.* Chicago: Health Administration Press.

Chapter 7   In a Few Words . . .

In excellent HCOs, nursing complements, supplements, and in some situations replaces physician care. Nurses have increasing responsibilities not only for acute care but also for primary, long-term, home, and palliative care. Supporting this role requires transformational leadership that focuses on meeting patients' plan-of-care needs and attracting nursing associates who want to continue to work and will encourage others to work for the organization. The nursing organization maintains infrastructure and processes for recruitment, functional protocols, professional development, and nurse satisfaction that meet those needs. The keys to success are the culture of empowerment, the measured performance, and the search for root causes to drive continuous improvement.

Nursing

Is This Your HCO?

Your HCO has "good but not great" measures in nursing quality, nurse satisfaction, and patient satisfaction. Your chief nursing officer (CNO) proposes that the hospital pursue Magnet Recognition Program status from the American Nurses Credentialing Center (ANCC). What should the senior management team think about?

1. Why pursue Magnet status? Probably not for the label. The payoff has to be in *your* mission achievement, not ANCC's. The fee should be justified by a substantial return in cost per case, via shorter stays, lower malpractice costs, and reduced turnover. How might that happen? The model is service excellence, tailored to nursing:

   Sound logistics, training, and supervision → *effective workers* → *higher performance.*

   The payoff comes via greater nurse satisfaction, greater patient satisfaction, greater physician satisfaction, and ultimately, increased market share.

2. Is there an alternative? Do-it-yourself is an alternative. What you get from the ANCC is tips, benchmarks, and discipline. You can reach Magnet performance without these by pursing nursing OFIs rigorously, but it might take longer.
3. Why not? The biggest reason is probably that your hospital is not ready yet in *sound logistics, training, and supervision.* "Magnet" makes a lot more sense when you've installed measured goals, built a reliable supply system, introduced formal training, helped your head nurses and supervisors learn transformational management, and celebrated some victories.

What to Do Next?

If clinical excellence were easy to achieve, more HCOs would be there. Where are the potholes on the path to perfection? Your coach says, "Keep a close eye out for the following":

- *Misunderstanding protocol application.* What a protocol does is put all team members on the same page. It only works when all associates know the protocol and are trained to implement it.
- *Under-using the interdisciplinary plan of care (IPOC).* No patient fits the protocol perfectly. The faster nurses and doctors identify the fit problems and address them, the faster the patient goes home. Each must make a professional evaluation, record it, and integrate his perspective with other team members.
- *Blocking and tackling failures.* The six nursing functions, shown in Exhibit 7.1, are summaries of a large number of clinical and managerial work processes. These are linked; when one fails, others are impaired. Measuring

them identifies OFIs. Addressing OFIs doesn't just fill the potholes; it rebuilds the highway.

- *Arguing over turf.* "Excellence in patient care" is the common ground. It makes you feel good, and it puts money in your pocket. Finding and agreeing on a solution that maximizes both feeling good and making money often takes time and energy, but it's worth it. Coaching, side conversations, visits to successful sites, scientific evidence, even a few deals are usually necessary. Process improvement teams (PITs) are where the conclusions are recorded. "Responsive listening" is where the progress is made.

In excellent HCOs, nursing complements, supplements, and in some situations replaces physician care. In all service lines, nursing adds a second diagnostic process and provides additional elements of care that are often critical to success. The nursing organization ensures that the nursing diagnosis and the additional elements of care are uniformly implemented for all patients across the HCO's spectrum of outpatient, inpatient, and continuing care.

This vision of nursing is a major redirection for many HCOs. Implementing it calls for a culture of empowerment, new approaches to the nursing role, expanded training for staff nurses and nurse managers, measured performance, and enhanced collaboration with physicians and other caregivers. When implementation is successful:

- All nursing associates are "delighted" with their work role.
- Staff turnover is less than 10 percent.
- All units deliver excellent care, as measured by outcomes, process quality, and HCAHPS patient satisfaction.

- Staffing is adequate to patient need, as documented by the measured outcomes.
- Functional protocols and training allow effective and increased use of less skilled nursing associates.
- Excellent nursing decreases complications, length of stay, readmissions, and malpractice risks. As a result, it contributes to healthy profit margins.

More than 300 HCOs have documented their success at this model through the American Nurses Credentialing Center's Magnet Recognition Program (www.nursecredentialing.org/Magnet.aspx). An unknown number of other HCOs have implemented the concepts independently.

The excellent nursing organization performs five functions, beginning with the provision of excellent patient care, as shown in Exhibit 7.1. Nursing must also coordinate all other care. It provides the majority of patient and family education and much of community health education. As the day-to-day leaders of most patient care teams, nurses must have managerial skills, including the ability to sustain the transformational environment, manage staff and resources, and provide for staff development. The nursing voice is critical on most planning committees, protocol selection committees, and PITs, and nurses are expected to improve their own performance.

HOW DOES AN HCO START THE MOVE TO EXCELLENT NURSING?

The transformational culture of empowerment and responsive management is the key to the transition. It makes the value of "respect" a reality; the condescension, sexism, evasion, and blaming common to authoritarian cultures become unacceptable. The steps outlined in Chapter 2 are the foundation for the transition. They have an immediate return in reduced turnover and a clearer

Exhibit 7.1 Nursing Functions

Function	Activities	Results
Deliver excellent care	Implement the nursing process: identify patients' needs, nursing diagnosis, and care plan.	Each patient has a nursing diagnosis and care plan.
	Integrate nursing process with IPOCs.	The plan is coordinated with patient management protocols and IPOCs.
	Coordinate IPOC implementation.	Progress toward maximal function is monitored.
	Evaluate patient progress.	Optimal outcomes are achieved for safe, effective, patient-centered, timely, efficient, and equitable care.
	Use case management for complicated cases.	
Coordinate and monitor interdisciplinary care	Communicate and integrate with physicians, other clinical support services (CSS), and other service lines.	Interdisciplinary patient rounds and IPOC used to coordinate care.
		Schedule coordinates diagnostic testing and therapeutic interventions.
	Pursue and correct gaps or problems in care management.	Patient and family needs for spiritual care, social services, palliative care, ethics consultation are identified and met.
Educate patients, families, and communities	Meet or exceed expectations of patients, other stakeholders.	Patient education materials
		Mentoring programs for new nurses
	Maintain professional nursing model and advancement in knowledge and skill-based competencies.	Management and leadership development programs
		Continuing education program (in house)
		Promotion of professional certification and advancement

Continued

Exhibit 7.1 Continued

Function	Activities	Results
Maintain the nursing organization	Project future personnel and facility needs; budget; ensure appropriate number and skill of staff complement. Recruit, select, retain, and motivate an effective workforce based on participation, HCO decision involvement, and empowerment.	Effective skill mix (RN, LPN, unlicensed assistive personnel, contract) and numbers of personnel to match patient needs Facility, equipment, and supply needs met
Improve nursing performance	Continuously improve nursing practice. Translate nursing research into practice improvements. Integrate organizational structures and management processes to plan and deliver nursing care. Inspire shared vision, commitment, creative responses to challenges.	Nursing practice councils for improvement, education, research, and standards Performance reviews Shared governance Competitive salaries and benefits Positive relationships established within HCO and community Budgets, facilities, equipment plans, emergency preparedness plans and drills, marketing strategies Leadership development plans

picture of the OFI agenda. Although the transition need not be perfect or universal, it is almost certainly inescapable: there are no documented cases of excellence under authoritarian cultures.

The transition requires new learning for many managers, including those in service lines, senior management, and nursing. The learning must be reinforced by modeling; it must be clear that older styles are no longer acceptable.

WHAT IS THE PROCESS BEHIND EXCELLENT NURSING CARE?

Nurses deliver excellent care using the nursing process, a comprehensive system of assessing, diagnosing, coordinating, implementing, and evaluating care. Exhibit 7.2 shows the elements of the nursing process with knowledge management resource requirements and examples. The process centers around a nursing care plan. The nursing care plan is a road map similar to the patient management protocol, but it emphasizes the patient's unique needs.

A good care plan does the following:

- Adapts the patient management protocol to the specific needs of the patient.
- Anticipates individual variations to prevent complications.
- Establishes a plan for nursing interventions. Patient-specific nursing treatments are defined and standardized by a Nursing Interventions Classification (NIC) list and may be classified according to 433 interventions.
- Organizes the major events in the hospitalization or disease episode to minimize overall duration.
- Establishes realistic clinical outcomes and a timetable for their achievement (Nursing Outcomes Classification [NOC] is a comprehensive, standardized classification of over 300 patient/client outcomes developed to evaluate the effects of nursing interventions).

Exhibit 7.2 Nursing Process Example for Airway Management

Elements of the Nursing Process	Resources and Guidelines	Examples
Assessment	Objective and subjective data	Vital signs, breath sounds, observation of difficulty breathing; laboratory results; physical examination
Nursing diagnosis	North American Nursing Diagnosis Association–International	Ineffective airway clearance related to tracheobronchial infection (pneumonia) and excess thick secretions as evidenced by abnormal breath sounds; crackles, wheezes; change in rate and depth of respiration; and effective cough with sputum.
Plan of care	Interdisciplinary plan of care	Effective airway clearance as evidenced by normal breath sounds; no crackles or wheezes; respiration rate 14–18 per minute; and no cough by within one week.
Implementation of care	Nursing Interventions Classification	Instruct and assist patient to TCDB (turn, cough, deep breathe) for assistance in loosening and expectorating mucus every two hours. A "rapid response team" is available if the patient's condition becomes life-threatening.
Evaluation of care	Nursing Outcomes Classification	Monitor improvements in breathing, expectorating mucus, and objective measures of oxygen profusion by physical examination and results of diagnostic tests; adjust goals, communicate with physician and CSS for modifications to patient management; provide education on stopping smoking, if applicable.

- Incorporates a discharge plan.
- Identifies potential barriers to prompt discharge, and how to investigate and remove them.

The nursing care plan is integrated into the interdisciplinary plan of care (IPOC). The timetable and advance planning on potential barriers are effective devices to reduce length of stay and cost per case.

The nursing process is a breakthrough advance. It identifies what needs to be done for each patient in terms that allow validation, measurement, and short-term forecasting. Picture any nursing setting, such as a clinic, an ICU, or a home care program. Five new and 15 return patients are expected. The workload for the new patients is clear; it is to establish the nursing process. The workload for the returning patients is specified in detail in the nursing interventions classifications (NICs), each of which is fully described in a functional protocol. The nursing outcomes classifications (NOCs) establish measurable goals at the patient level. Of course, emergencies will arise, and the specifics will be radically different in each setting, but the nursing process establishes several elements critical to the effective operation of the units:

- Nursing contributions to the IPOC. These improve the patient's response by identifying and addressing emotional, social, and environmental concomitants of disease and treatment.
- The tasks that must be performed. These are specified in functional protocols.
- The time required to complete these tasks, by associate skill level. The protocols have requirements for the minimum acceptable professional level and task-specific certification.
- The minimum staffing requirement, by professional level, and an estimate of total nursing staff required.

- The requirements for coordination of clinical support services.
- The logistic requirements for supplies, equipment, and facilities.
- A classification system that supports measurement of performance. The nursing and medical diagnoses provide the specification necessary to use process measures of care and, as a second step, relate these to outcomes. The functional and patient management protocols provide the quality measures themselves.

In short, the process establishes a reliable forecast of what needs to be done, what resources are needed to do it, and how the results can be measured. Because it is founded in a classification system, any care plan can be audited and tested by a competent professional. Alternatives can be evaluated. Ultimately, each NIC can be scientifically studied in terms of its contribution to excellent care.

What is described above is evidence-based nursing for the 21st century. It is a vision that is probably not fully achieved today at any HCO, but it will be realized, and excellent HCOs are further down the path than "pretty good" ones.

WHAT ARE THE CLINICAL IMPLICATIONS OF 21ST CENTURY NURSING?

The nursing process approach expands and improves clinical care in two major ways:

1. The emphasis on emotional, social, and environmental factors identifies and removes elements that contribute to complications, delays, and treatment failures.
2. Predictability means the right care is on hand, on time, and effectively delivered.

The patients' chance of recovery, extent of recovery, and speed of recovery are improved, and the cost of care is reduced.

Dealing with emotional, social, and environmental factors requires expanded services. Expert consultation on inter-current disease, diet, ethics, and controllable risk factors is frequently necessary. Patient training and support programs are required. Post-discharge follow-up is often essential. Home and continuing care services must be improved. These call for new services in many HCOs. The full pattern of excellence—the optimal service design for small, medium, and large communities—remains to be developed, but the picture of increased coordination and a continuing clinical responsibility is clear.

HOW DOES NURSING MANAGE THE IPOC?

Nurses generally coordinate and monitor progress throughout the episode of care, whether it is in an inpatient, outpatient, or home setting. The goal is to organize all elements of care in the most patient-satisfactory and least costly elapsed time. The IPOC guides sequencing and scheduling diagnostic and treatment interventions (including transportation) and monitoring for irregularities in logistics and patients' responses to interventions. It is increasingly computerized. It is accessible to all caregivers. In intensive care, much data are entered from monitoring machines. The IPOC must include symptoms and complaints, concurrent disease or complications, working diagnosis, and medical orders and the nursing care plan. It must also include safety alerts, such as patient allergies and language barriers.

The nursing team is responsible for the following kinds of monitoring activities:

• Ensuring that the patient's physician has completed diagnosis, treatment, and appropriate follow-up activities in an appropriate and timely manner

- Reporting clinical observations to the physician and other members of the caregiving team
- Identifying progress of patient goals as identified in the IPOC
- Assessing and reporting relevant psychosocial and family-related factors
- Assessing effectiveness of nursing interventions
- Knowing where patients are, and receiving them from clinical support services (CSS)
- Receiving and transmitting results of reports from CSS
- Preparing and forwarding unexpected events reports

The nurse as a patient advocate is expected to take appropriate action diplomatically and effectively. Nurses catch omitted, wrong, lost, conflicting, and delayed reports and orders on a daily basis. They are the first to see unexpected results and unsatisfactory treatments. They remind, persuade, cajole, and convince others to correct these problems quickly so that they do not escalate. The transformational culture makes it possible for them to do this comfortably.

WHAT ARE THE OPERATIONAL IMPLICATIONS OF 21ST CENTURY NURSING?

It is probably impossible to make the transition to nursing excellence in the absence of the cultural and operations support of an effective HCO.

The operational agenda for excellence is clear:

- Service lines
- Responsive leadership
- Knowledge management
- Clinical and managerial training

- Safe, effective, attractive environment of care
- Funds for appropriate equipment
- Supplies

These bedside and examining room essentials must be backed by:

- Continuous improvement
- Marketing
- Strategic management

That is to say, excellent nursing requires an excellent HCO. And vice versa.

HOW DOES NURSING SUSTAIN THE TRANSFORMATIONAL CULTURE?

Nurse managers are expected to implement the transformational culture described in Chapter 2. Each nurse manager must be specifically trained in transformational management: how to encourage associates, respond to recurring questions, implement process and protocol changes, and celebrate gains. Because success often involves interdisciplinary collaboration, nurse managers must be proficient in teamwork, mediation, and consensus building.

These skills are taught through programs in human resources management. Leading HCOs back up formal education with responsive listening by superiors and senior management. They routinely assign coaches and mentors to new nurse managers and use a mentoring system to develop new staff nurses. They use 360-degree surveys to give nurse managers comprehensive assessment. They provide personal development programs for nurses and nurse managers and carefully monitor the nurse managers' satisfaction.

WHAT IS THE KEY TO "NO NURSING SHORTAGE"?

Adequate nurse staffing is tailored to the specific needs of each unit, based on factors including patient acuity, the experience of the nursing staff, the skill mix of the staff, available technology, and the support services available to nurses. Although California has mandated minimum nurse staffing levels since 2004 and other states have attempted to follow suit, there is little evidence that regulatory approaches are effective in improving quality.

Adequate staffing achieves two goals:

1. Measured quality of patient care and patient satisfaction meet or approach benchmark.
2. Nursing associates are "delighted" with their work setting, as measured by satisfaction surveys, turnover, and absenteeism.

Attaining adequate staffing goes well beyond specific numbers of personnel per patient. Most important in developing a long-term solution is to involve the unit nurses in the staffing and scheduling decisions. Because "delighting" them is an explicit goal, they are empowered to determine the staffing. The organization's role is to help them get the minimum acceptable staffing. Exhibit 7.3 shows the seven levels of response.

The failure of many earlier "staffing models" was certainly related to their authoritarian imposition. They set the unit's staff in the front office, not in negotiation with the staff itself. The failure was almost certainly also related to lack of comprehensiveness. One activity or a few were used where all were required. Here are some of the important issues by level:

1. Average and peak needs: Many units are quite stable from shift to shift, and it is easy to establish a minimum requirement based on fulfilling patient needs. Others are highly

Exhibit 7.3 Responses to Variability in Nurse Staffing Needs

Application	Activity	Examples
All units	Average and peak staff needs are established from records of past patients	Historic "feel" for adequate staff Study of inter-shift variability Analysis of specific work requirements by actual tasks required by patients
	Review of quality and patient and physician satisfaction outcomes	Ongoing achievement of outcomes and process quality goals OFIs for improving patient care
	Reliance on "extra effort"	Brief intervals of staff shortages or high patient demand
	Review of nursing associate satisfaction	OFIs for improving work environment
High-variability units	Control of patient flow	Patient scheduling Diversion of patients
	Scheduling and overtime	Flexible schedules and advance notice of workload Associate-requested overtime Occasional and negotiated overtime
	Trained supplementary associates	Part-time on-call associates "Relief" associates from a specially trained and compensated pool

variable. The IPOC and functional protocols introduce new understanding of what must be done, who must do it, and how long it takes. This makes it easier to establish the minimum, and also to collect data and understand the variability.

2. Any failure of a patient quality goal or a failure in physician satisfaction is a high-priority OFI. Study of root causes can open important avenues: more efficient protocols, better training, and alternative solutions. This ongoing study simultaneously improves efficiency. The work output per associate should increase over time.

3. All humans are capable of extra effort. Most work situations require it, and most associates expect it. Many associates seek overtime and are happy to respond. If the base staffing is adequate, extra effort provides the first solution to variability, one that is adequate in many nursing settings. Two limits must be carefully observed:

   a. Individuals are never asked for more than they can safely and effectively deliver.

   b. The overload situation is the exception, not the routine.

4. The second test of an effective program is associate satisfaction. A well-designed system will routinely pass both patient care and associate tests.

5. Patient scheduling is often an effective response. Most medical care needs are not life-threatening. Scheduling them in advance reduces workload variation. Occasional rescheduling when other emergencies intervene does not impair patient care goals and avoids associate overloads. ICUs, EDs, and OB units are exceptions, because the demand cannot safely be scheduled.

6. Predictable work schedules are known to be important, as is the ability to request time off in advance or arrange specific shifts or hours. Electronic scheduling systems fulfill all of these criteria.

7. Where all else fails, the HCO must provide effective staff supplementation. This is not "agency nurses." It is a cadre

of specially trained, additionally compensated associates who know the unit and its patients' needs and can move in on short notice.

CAN NURSING IMPROVE PERFORMANCE?

All nursing teams are responsible for maintaining the transformational culture and for improving unit performance. They monitor the operating scorecard of their unit, as described below. They are actively supported by the nursing organization and senior management, who are frequent visitors and responsive listeners. The nursing organization includes clinical specialists who can assist with nursing process issues. Under this system, each team has support for any kind of problem, as shown in Exhibit 7.4.

HOW CAN YOU MEASURE NURSING?

The combined developments of evidence-based medicine, electronic information management, and the Nursing Outcomes Classification (NOC) have made it feasible to measure performance of most nursing teams. The array of data will provide increasingly valuable answers to core nursing questions about best practice, staffing levels, and training methods. The National Quality Forum has developed 15 standards for nursing-sensitive care for which additional data may need to be collected. Examples are shown in Exhibit 7.5.

Exhibit 7.4 Assistance Available to Nursing Teams

In all of these examples, an unanswered need can be reported either to the nursing organization or senior management, who are expected to correct the problem and eliminate recurrence.

Kind of Problem	Support Available
Difficulty with functional or patient management protocol	All protocols are subject to revision when necessary. Training may be the solution for individual issues.
Equipment, supply, or facilities failure	Plant services associates are trained to respond promptly. Their operating scorecards assess delays and nurse satisfaction.
Personal difficulty of team member	Human resources management has counseling and retraining services.
Harassment or inappropriate behavior toward a team member	Harassment is defined by the associates. Human resources management, the nursing organization, and senior management are trained in effective responses.
Staffing shortage	The nursing organization is committed to effective staffing. A process improvement team (PIT) will address ways to improve staff productivity, reduce variability in patient demand, or revise staffing.
Unexpected clinical event	Reporting is mandatory. The unit team is trained to make an emergency response. It may participate in service recovery, further analysis, or a PIT addressing risk management.
Unexpected customer or associate event	The unit team is expected to pursue appropriate service recovery, emergency response, and reporting for review of trends. Reporting is mandatory.

Exhibit 7.5 Nursing Performance Measures

Dimension	Inpatient Examples	Outpatient Examples (Home Care Program)	Community Nursing Examples
Demand	Number and acuity of patients, percent emergencies	Scheduled home visits, delay for visit	Enrollment in programs, percent eligibles attracted
Costs	Nursing hours per patient day,* medical supplies	Payroll costs, home supplies, travel costs	Faculty cost, facility cost, promotional cost
Human resources	Skills mix, education and certification,** nurse satisfaction, ** turnover, vacancies	Skill mix, satisfaction, turnover, vacancies	Skill mix, satisfaction, turnover, vacancies
Output/productivity	Discharges, cost per discharge, cost per member month	Visits, visits per patient, patients per visiting nurse, costs per patient month	Number of presentations, attendance, cost per member
Outcomes/quality	Falls prevalence,* urinary tract infections,* ventilator-associated pneumonia,* pressure ulcer prevalence*	Daily living scores, hospitalizations, transfers to long-term care	Percent members smoking, percent seeking prenatal care, child trauma

Continued

Exhibit 7.5 Continued

Dimension	Inpatient Examples	Outpatient Examples (Home Care Program)	Community Nursing Examples
Process quality	Percent complete care plans, medication errors, percent presurgery patient education, pain assessment**	Percent visits late or missed, errors in equipment, supplies	Member awareness, curriculum evaluation, facility evaluation
Patient satisfaction	Percent "very satisfied," number of complaints	Percent "very satisfied," family satisfaction	Audience evaluation, member satisfaction
Physician satisfaction	Percent of referring physicians and attending physicians "very satisfied," complaints	Percent of referring physicians "very satisfied," complaints	Physician awareness, satisfaction, complaints

*Endorsed by the National Quality Forum (NQF) as National Voluntary Consensus Standards for Nursing-Sensitive Care. For a complete list of NQF-endorsed nursing-sensitive standards, see NQF's National Voluntary Consensus Standards for Nursing-Sensitive Care. Washington, DC: NQF. Available at www.qualityforum.org.
** Included in the American Nursing Association (ANA) National Database of Nursing Quality Indicators. For a list of the indicators, see ANA's National Database of Nursing Quality Indicators. Silver Spring, MD: ANA. Available at www.nursingquality.org/.

SUGGESTED READINGS

American Nurses Association. 2009. *Nursing Administration: Scope and Standards of Practice.* Silver Spring, MD: American Nurses Association.

Bulechek, G. M., H. K. Butcher, and J. M. Dochterman. 2007. *Nursing Interventions Classification,* 5th edition. St. Louis, MO: Mosby.

Lindberg, C., S. Nash, and C. Lindberg. 2008. *On the Edge: Nursing in the Age of Complexity.* Bordentown, NJ: Plexus Press.

Powell, S. K., and H. A. Tahan. 2009. *Case Management: A Practical Guide for Education and Practice,* 3rd edition. Philadelphia, PA: Lippincott Williams & Wilkins.

Sullivan, E. J. 2008. *Effective Leadership and Management in Nursing,* 7th edition. Upper Saddle River, NJ: Pearson Prentice Hall.

Swanson, E., S. Moorhead, M. Johnson, and M. L. Maas. 2007. *Nursing Outcomes Classification,* 4th edition. St. Louis, MO: Mosby.

Chapter 8 In a Few Words . . .

Most seriously ill patients require several clinical support services (CSS). Most CSS can exist independently, but their collective, integrated availability is a core contribution of the modern HCO. The HCO's role is to ensure safe, effective, patient-centered, timely, efficient, and equitable care, providing comprehensive and integrated one-stop shopping that is superior to service offered by independent providers. To do this, the HCO must first create an environment where qualified CSS professionals and other associates want to work. Then it supports the CSS to achieve excellence within its domain. The HCO provides a stable market for CSS and integrates them into overall clinical excellence. It also often provides information management, training and personnel services, physical facilities, and strategic guidance. A culture of empowerment, measured performance, annual goals, and continuous improvement are required for a successful relationship.

Clinical Support
Services

Is This Your HCO?

You have operational measures (Exhibit 8.4) in place for every CSS. Performance is "pretty good" and in some cases much better than that. Quality and patient satisfaction measures tend to be better than cost and caregiver satisfaction measures. CSS are rarely a big problem to caregivers, but there are so many CSS, and they provide so much service, that there is always an undercurrent of difficulties.

Building an excellent relationship starts with the HCO's obligations to each CSS, exhibits 8.1 and 8.2. The HCO controls the overall size; it must check its plan annually. The HCO provides a broad spectrum of space, supplies, funds, and training; those services should push benchmark (chapters 11 and 12). The HCO coordinates services; the CSS must be involved in every relevant process improvement team (PIT). The HCO generates markets; these should be robust.

When the HCO meets its obligations, it's hard for the CSS to walk away. The negotiation should be around the specific opportunities for improvement (OFIs)—places where measured performance can clearly be improved. "How can we help you move to benchmark?" is the opening question.

Behind it lies the reality that CSS associates' incomes will improve as benchmark is reached. The HCO should stimulate clinical PITs and bear the cost of running them (it's peanuts). The HCO should have the training programs to implement change and the capital to meet improvement needs.

What to Do Next?

What if a CSS doesn't respond when HCO support is adequate and incentives are in place? It happens, even with complex professional CSS like pathology. What's the right stance?

Your coach says:

1. How much is it worth to fix it? Opportunities that directly affect cost per case, length of stay, and market share can be worth a lot. Small stuff is exactly that.

2. Almost all CSS are now commodities. If you don't get what you need from your team, there are many competitors willing to take the business on competitive terms, even in pathology, imaging, and pharmacy. The CSS should be reminded of that, as politely as possible.

3. The first option is always to help the current team move to benchmark. The HCO's loyalty to a CSS team is important. But with repeated failure to match the documented performance of other HCOs, the contract should not be renewed. What's happening is that a small group of associates are hampering the majority of stakeholders, including patients and caregivers alike. That's intolerable.

Caregiving requires services from dozens of specialized professionals providing important diagnostic information (e.g., laboratory, imaging, electrophysiology) or therapeutic interventions (e.g., pharmacy, surgical facilities, social services, pastoral care, ethics committees, health education). Each clinical support service (CSS) has its own technology and procedures discussed extensively in its professional literature. CSS are ordered by an attending physician or nurse based on the patient management protocol or interdisciplinary plan of care (IPOC). A serious illness may require several hundred interventions, involving a dozen or more CSS at several sites—outpatient offices, the acute care hospital, long-term care facilities, and home.

The purpose of any CSS is to:

provide its specialized services at a level that is clinically excellent and meets patients' and caregivers' needs for service.

The purpose of the HCO is to assist each CSS in achieving its purpose, and also to:

provide a set of CSS that optimally meets community need.

The HCO's purpose implies that the profile of available CSS must be consistent with the strategic plan, but for most HCOs it also implies that some patients must be referred for some CSS; "optimal" is not "all." The HCO's competitive advantage is its ability to integrate the package for each patient's needs, fulfilling in total the goal of safe, effective, patient-centered, timely, efficient, and equitable care. The quality, cost, amenities, and effective use of each CSS are directly related to overall HCO mission achievement.

WHAT'S THE CORE CSS-HCO RELATIONSHIP?

The HCO contracts with each CSS, selecting one of several forms for the contract, including employment, strategic partnerships, joint ventures, and corporate subsidiaries. In many cases, the HCO has a choice of alternatives. For example, imaging and pharmacy are offered as contract services as well as through more conventional structures. At least theoretically, the HCO can buy imaging as it buys laundry service, or it could employ radiologists and the entire imaging service. While the forms vary, the underlying goals of the contract remain the same. Exhibit 8.1 outlines the major elements that each CSS contract must address. The foundation of a sound relationship is the thorough and accurate specification of each of these elements.

Contracts in excellent HCOs are good-faith collaborations rather than adversarial negotiations. The goal is to meet the needs of all parties—patients' needs first, but also the needs of physicians and nurses, the HCO, the community, and CSS associates. Viewing the CSS from this perspective makes clear that the relationship is a partnership where both parties are empowered, and it helps make clear the rights and duties of each partner. The balance of this chapter's questions address implementing the contract elements.

HOW DOES THE HCO FULFILL THE CONTRACT?

The HCO keeps the contracts collaborative by responsive listening, fulfilling its obligations to the CSS, and providing for CSS needs in a way that makes the relationship "a great place to give care." CSS associates, whether employed or contracted, have similar privileges and obligations to other associates and are not treated any differently. They must respect the values, complete the general training, follow the rules, and participate in the celebrations. Their goals tie them to the common mission, and as

Exhibit 8.1 Core Elements of CSS-HCO Contracts

Element	Definition	Contribution
Patient care objective	Scope, size, location, and hours of services to be provided	The contribution of the CSS to excellent care is described clearly for both customer and associate audiences.
		The HCO negotiates size, scope, and hours.
Standard of performance	Operational performance measures	The measures for the six operational dimensions are established, with benchmarks and acceptable minimums.
Compliance with mission, vision, and values	CSS managers and associates share commitment of other associates	CSS associates are equal-rights and equal-obligations team members with other associates.
Credentialing	Certifications and performance standard for individuals	CSS associates meet equivalent standards of professional conduct and performance.
Commitment to continuous improvement	Annual goal-negotiating process, participation in PITs	CSS is committed to participate with other associates in process improvement.

Continued

Exhibit 8.1 Continued

Element	Definition	Contribution
HCO contribution	Services supplied by the HCO	HCO provides logistic and strategic services, including audit, to agreed-upon performance measures.
		HCO is also responsible for helping CSS integrate with other CSS and service lines.
Compensation	Financial arrangements	Sources of funds, accounting services, limitations on commitments, and incentive compensation arrangements are agreed upon.
Competitive restriction	Limitations on CSS rights to offer competing services	HCO protects against independent competition by the CSS.
Renewal/termination	Opportunities to re-open, renew, or terminate contract	HCO protects against major failure of CSS.

improvement occurs, they receive appropriate rewards. The annual goal-setting is a joint exploration of OFIs and a shared plan to achieve them. In short, the contract assumes CSS associates are part of the HCO, sharing its mission, its transformational culture, and its evidence-based management.

Each CSS must have a clear line of accountability to the governing board. A designated manager (the post can have a variety of titles) employed by the HCO must manage this accountability, making sure that patients' needs, other caregivers' needs, and CSS associates' needs are identified and met.

HOW DOES THE CSS FULFILL THE CONTRACT?

CSS have very different characteristics, yet similarities emerge at one level of abstraction above these differences. Social service and radiation therapy, for example, share common functions identified in Exhibit 8.2.

WHY DOES THE HCO NEGOTIATE THE AVAILABILITY OF EACH CSS?

The contract specifies the size, locations, and hours of service of each CSS. The HCO uses its epidemiologic planning model to forecast demand. Patient need and convenience must be balanced against volume to ensure acceptable provider skills and operating costs. Use must be limited to clinically appropriate cases. Benchmarks for CSS quality and cost per unit of service provide practical guidelines for planning and operations. By contracting with large referral centers, even the smallest HCO can arrange to meet any patient's need and provide as much convenience as the local demand will support.

Final control of availability rests with the HCO's governing board. In return for that control, the HCO must ensure competitive

Exhibit 8.2 Functions of CSS, Showing Service and HCO Roles

Function	CSS Role	HCO Role
Provide excellent care	Select, use, maintain, and teach functional protocols. Participate in patient management protocol selection and development.	Assist in designing work processes and training programs. Ensure appropriate voice in patient management protocol selection committees. Maintain a central scheduling system.
Maintain patient relationships	Schedule patients effectively. Train associates in identifying patient needs and using techniques to improve acceptability of care. Maintain cultural competence. Provide for uninsured patients.	Provide associate sensitivity training. Provide translators and cultural competence training. Recognize burden of non-paying patients in contract.
Maintain consultative relationships	Assist caregivers with protocol administration. Consult on questionable cases. Provide training to other professions on advances in their CSS.	Support CSS involvement in PITs and planning activities. Incorporate consultation and training into contract. Resolve rules for non-professional administration of CSS services.
Plan and manage operations	Negotiate appropriate long-term relationships. Negotiate goals for operational scorecard dimensions.	Negotiate appropriate long-term relationships. Establish compensation and contribution from HCO's annual strategic goals.
Promote continuous improvement of service	Benchmark, identify OFIs, and establish and participate in PITs.	Negotiate, support, and reward improvement.

income and attractive working conditions for CSS associates. CSS contracts limit direct competitive activity; the HCO's laboratory has specific limits on its ability to sell services to HCO physicians in private practice.

WHAT ARE THE ELEMENTS OF EXCELLENT CSS CARE?

Each CSS must be led by an appropriately trained and credentialed professional who maintains measured performance, establishes OFIs, and moves toward benchmark. But excellence also requires the careful integration of CSS into each patient's IPOC. CSS must participate in the performance improvement of most service lines, and must collaborate with other CSS on a regular basis. They do this through the following mechanisms.

1. *Patient management protocols:* These specify when CSS are required, optional, and not recommended. As a result, they also control the demand for service. CSS members participate actively in protocol selection committees.

2. *Functional protocols:* Virtually all CSS activities are learned processes that are recorded as functional protocols reflecting best practice for the CSS profession. Each CSS designs, tests, and maintains the processes it uses, its performance measures, and its benchmarks. These are included in the contract and drive the continuous improvement process. Many functional protocols must be integrated across several CSS and nursing. Integration is achieved by PITs that include all units involved.

3. *Scheduling systems:* Timely patient service must be balanced against an orderly workflow within the CSS. Sophisticated scheduling systems achieve this by managing the demand stream. The best scheduling systems integrate all CSS to minimize the length of the patient care event.

4. *Training:* Each CSS must rely on a mix of professional and non-professional associates. Maximizing the contribution of non-professionals is important to improve safety, patient-centeredness, and costs. It is achieved by careful training and transformational supervision. The HCO provides training in supervision and continuous improvement, cultural competence, and other issues shared by several CSS. The CSS supplies training for its functional protocols, but often collaborates with human resources management to implement and evaluate the training.

The HCO Performance Improvement Council (PIC) uses PITs and planning committees to negotiate questions ranging from coordination and availability of services (will Imaging have full service 24/7? what arrangements exist for inpatient meals delayed by testing?), to coverage of uninsured patients (who pays the rehabilitation costs for an uninsured trauma patient?), to privileges for specific CSS assigned to various associate groups (will images taken in outpatient offices be included in the medical record, and which will be read by the imagist?).

WHAT DRIVES A GOOD CLINICAL SCHEDULING SYSTEM?

The scheduling system is challenging for all HCOs. It arranges the location of care (e.g., ED to inpatient, outpatient surgery, or clinic visits) and the CSS. Patient needs require attention to safety, satisfaction, and efficiency. CSS delays often add to the total length of stay and increase the cost per case. The CSS and nursing units need a manageable workflow. Associates need planned schedules, but they also need work. Idle time drives up the cost per test and reduces associates' skills.

The concept for the scheduling system is shown in Exhibit 8.3. Unless volumes of work are large (laboratory and pharmacy,

Exhibit 8.3 Conceptual Model of Sophisticated Scheduling Process

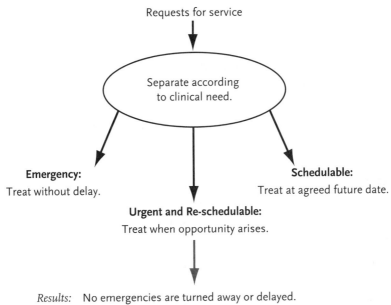

Requests for service

Separate according to clinical need.

Emergency:
Treat without delay.

Urgent and Re-schedulable:
Treat when opportunity arises.

Schedulable:
Treat at agreed future date.

Results: No emergencies are turned away or delayed.
More urgent and schedulable patients are seen sooner.
Patients seeking fixed date get a fixed date.
CSS efficiency (cases per associate or cost per test or treatment) increases.

for example), a CSS or a nursing unit that simply accepts patients as they come will have periodic idle times and overflow demand. The first wastes money; the second endangers safety and satisfaction. Sophisticated scheduling systems can substantially reduce both problems. The secret is to identify some set of patients who do not have emergency needs and are willing and able to come on call. Non-emergency patients already in the HCO are an example. As the exhibit shows, emergency patients get immediate care. On-call patients get a fixed future date, but they also can be called sooner. Scheduled patients get a fixed future date. At a given level of emergency allowance, overall efficiency will increase and overall delays will decrease by calling in patients.

Sophisticated computerized scheduling systems are available for major support services and for admission and occupancy management. Most scheduling systems can also be operated in a simulation mode to analyze the costs and benefits of alternative strategies. Simulation outputs are useful in both short- and long-term planning to evaluate potential improvements in demand categorization, resource availability, and scheduling rules.

WHO ARE CSS CUSTOMERS?

CSS must view both caregivers and patients as customers, and recognize that caregivers often have competitive alternatives. To win the orders, CSS must meet caregiver needs:

- Excellent care: Errors, unexpected events, and patient dissatisfaction are near zero.
- Consultative advice: Each CSS is an expert resource. Caregivers should be encouraged to seek advice in properly using CSS resources.
- Protocol improvement: Many questions that arise in the adoption of guidelines require CSS participation to answer. Most protocols must be agreed to by the CSS involved.
- Training: CSS advances can change how care is given. Many procedures originated in CSS but have moved to general usage; caregivers must often be trained to do them. Others have complex implications for other parts of care, and caregivers must be trained to understand those interactions.
- Assistance with uninsured patients: The plans must be worked out in advance and specified in the contract with the HCO.

These needs are met by CSS participation in PITs and planning committees and support of training activities. Participation must be negotiated in the CSS-HCO contract.

CAN THE HCO ENSURE COMPETITIVE INCOMES FOR CSS ASSOCIATES?

The HCO controls a lucrative stream of business for each CSS, but that does not automatically ensure each associate has competitive compensation. Competitive compensation does not mean "As much as you can earn someplace else," because the HCO will expect care limited to appropriateness standards and assigned to the lowest capable level of worker. It means "As much as you could earn someplace else *given that you accept our commitment to mission and evidence-based medicine.*" Perverse incentives of the payment system complicate implementing that definition. Income for the HCO and the CSS are at stake, but income for both must be secondary to the mission. Sound solutions require adhering to principles of evidence-based medicine and management, solid analysis of the market situation, and a robust negotiating process. The HCO must be scrupulous in its commitment to mission, but at the same time assure both itself and the CSS associates of a competitive income opportunity.

Excellent HCOs implement that approach using a four-part strategy. First, the CSS must be carefully sized to realistic market needs using the epidemiologic planning model. The model forecasts demand and income for individual professionals. Second, the HCO must implement a transformational culture to make the work attractive to professional and non-professional associates. Third, the HCO performance must approach benchmark in all the logistic and strategic services the CSS needs. Fourth, the contract must be competitive in the CSS associates' eyes. HCOs that have implemented this approach are prepared for payment system revisions such as bundled payments.

HOW ARE ANNUAL GOALS NEGOTIATED?

Measures, benchmarks, OFIs, improved goals, and rewards should be routine in all CSS. For CSS where the HCO provides some or all capital, there are two interrelated negotiations: setting annual operating goals and identifying and justifying new capital investment.

A unit that has been diligent in the preceding year will be able to formulate next year's budget quickly, drawing in large part on work that has already been done in continuous improvement. Quality, costs, patient satisfaction, and associate satisfaction must be based on benchmarks; the management of a CSS that cannot meet benchmarks can usually be replaced by competitors with proven records. Well-run organizations have clearly defined budget process roles for the CSS manager, the budget manager (a technical support person or office attached to finance), and the HCO manager. The CSS manager and team are expected to:

- review the demand forecasts prepared by the budget manager, extending them to the specific levels required in the department and suggesting modifications based on their knowledge of the local situation;
- identify changes in the scope of services and the operating budget arising from changes in demand, new technology, patient management protocol development, and continuous improvement. Minor changes are incorporated in the operating budget. Major ones are addressed in the capital and new programs budget, discussed below;
- propose expectations for staffing, labor productivity, and supplies consistent with demand forecasts and constraints;
- propose goals in the operational scorecard measures for quality and satisfaction, using benchmark and available competitor data; and

- identify OFIs and initiatives that should be developed during the coming year.

The budget manager (Chapter 13) is expected to:

- assemble historical data on achievement of last year's budget;
- prepare forecasts of major CSS demand measures;
- prepare benchmark and competitor data;
- promulgate the budget guidelines for changes in total expenditures, profit, and capital investment approved by the finance committee of the board;
- circulate wage-increase guidelines from human resources and supplies-price guidelines from materials management;
- assist in calculations and prepare trial budgets until a satisfactory proposal for the board has been reached.

The HCO manager responsible for the CSS is expected to:

- ensure that the proposed goals do not impair quality or satisfaction in other units;
- assist the CSS and encourage steady but realistic improvement;
- coordinate interdepartmental issues that arise from the budgeting process;
- meet the budget guidelines set by the governing board or the senior management team;
- resolve conflicting needs among CSS;
- evaluate the progress of the CSS to assist in the distribution of incentives; and
- assist the CSS in pursuing OFIs and implementing them during the coming year.

CSS managers are responsible for identifying capital investment opportunities and developing specific proposals for new or replacement capital equipment or major revisions to service—called "programmatic proposals." Programmatic proposals are subject to a competitive review process that places them in rank order for board action (see Chapter 14). The investment will be justified by improvements in operational performance measures. If the proposal is accepted, the CSS will be expected to adopt and achieve those goals. Many benefits occur outside the CSS, making the collaborative approach to proposal development essential and committing the HCO to the future goals.

WHAT ARE THE CSS OPERATIONAL MEASURES?

Exhibit 8.4 summarizes measures appropriate for any CSS. Even the smallest CSS should have measures, benchmarks, OFIs, and annual improvement goals. Large, complex CSS will have a substantial measurement set, befitting their status as multi-million dollar enterprises. The HCO manager's focus should be on the aggregate performance, which should be routinely compared to benchmark and competitor values.

Most CSS quality measures are intermediate outcome or process compliance measures. In intermediate outcomes, follow-up inspection or similar assessment reveals that the CSS activity was or was not correctly performed and yielded the right information for further treatment. In process compliance, the inspection shows that the functional protocol was or was not followed. The two approaches provide in-depth understanding that identifies OFIs and facilitates their correction. Pathology laboratories have pursued these measures successfully, allowing them to ensure accuracy of their diagnostic reports. The College of American Pathologists maintains libraries of measures, values,

Exhibit 8.4 Performance Measures for CSS

Dimension	Measures	Applications
Demand	Requests for service	Used to forecast staff and other resource needs
		Specified by time, location, kind of service, and urgency of demand
	Market share	Used to track competitive success
		Specified by competitor and service if available
Costs	Fixed, variable, direct, and indirect costs	Used to analyze and improve work processes
	Physical units of resources	Resource use is specified by time, location, kind of service
	Age and repair records of equipment	Equipment records trigger maintenance and replacement
Human resources	Retention, absenteeism, injuries, satisfaction, recruitment, and training statistics	Used to ensure "a great place to give care"
		Specified by worker

Continued

Exhibit 8.4 *Continued*

Dimension	Measures	Applications
Output and productivity	Units of demand met and not met	Used to identify service failures
	Cost per unit of output	Used to benchmark efficiency
	Physical units consumed per unit of output	Specified by time, location, kind of service
Quality	Process compliance scores	Used to ensure compliance with functional protocols
	Unexpected event counts	Specified by time, location, kind of service
		Unexpected events are 100% investigated
Patient satisfaction	Overall satisfaction and specifics of service	Used to ensure favorable patient reaction
		Specified by time, location, kind of service
Physician satisfaction	Overall satisfaction and specifics of service	Used to ensure favorable referring physician satisfaction
		Specified by physician and patient groups

and education programs[1] and insists upon statistically controlled intermediate outcomes for accreditation.[2]

WHAT FORM OF AFFILIATION BEST MEETS THE HCO'S NEEDS?

The best CSS affiliation offers long-term performance closest to benchmark. The preferred solution is probably ownership; the HCO has ultimate control of employment, privileging, capital, protocol selection, training, location, and operating performance measures. Alternatives to ownership might be selected to facilitate associate incentives, to reduce capital costs, or to take advantage of skills developed through horizontal integration. A small number of commercial companies have offered CSS management services. Unlike the record in environment-of-care services, where outsourcing is the rule (see Chapter 12), it appears that few have captured substantial market share. Successful models include pharmacy services, some imaging services, and long-term acute care.

WHO CAN IMPLEMENT A CSS FUNCTIONAL PROTOCOL?

The criterion for the level of skill and training necessary to provide a given test or treatment is straightforward: it should normally be assigned to the lowest cost associate who is capable

---

[1] College of American Pathologists. [Online information; retrieved 10/15/09.] www.cap.org/apps/cap.portal?_nfpb=true&_pageLabel=home.

[2] College of American Pathologists, Commission on Laboratory Accreditation "Laboratory Accreditation Program Sample Checklist." [Online information; retrieved 10/15/09.] www.cap.org/apps/docs/laboratory_accreditation/ sample_checklist.pdf.

of maintaining quality and patient satisfaction standards, and available to all others who can maintain the standards.

Applying the criterion is a challenge. Definitive studies are rare. Standards of practice, a less rigorous level of evidence, are acceptable. If orthopedists and cardiologists elsewhere are privileged to act upon their own interpretation of images, they should be allowed to do that in our HCO. If a technician can prepare an echocardiogram at the Johns Hopkins Hospital, the task can be assigned to technicians at other HCOs *if they are trained and monitored as well as the Hopkins technician is trained and monitored.*

Application of the criterion should be assigned to medical staff protocol committees and PITs that can assemble evidence and recommend the safe but cost-effective solution. The committees and PITs must be guided to work from evidence rather than authority. The solution often is to permit lower skilled associates to proceed in uncomplicated cases, review the evidence emerging, and broaden their assignment as their record of success grows.

WHAT IS THE ROLE OF THE HCO MANAGER?

The HCO manager facilitates all the interactions shown in Exhibit 8.5. Here's a summary of the duties described above and normally arising from the ongoing relationship:

1. "Responsive listening," including frequent rounding, talking with associates in the CSS at all levels, and addressing their needs
2. Communicating information about and explanation of strategic guidelines, other relevant board decisions, OFIs and matters of interest arising from various surveillance activities, PIC actions, and the work of PITs potentially impacting the CSS

Exhibit 8.5 Core Organization of CSS

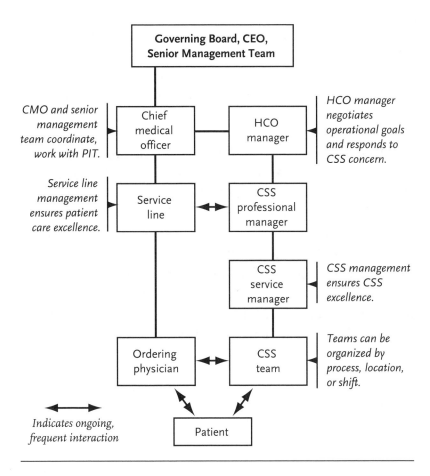

3. Supporting the CSS's PITs with assistance from clinical units and logistic and strategic services
4. Ensuring representation on all PITs directly impacting the CSS
5. Negotiating the annual operational goals—relating the CSS's improvement possibilities to needs of other units and identifying and resolving issues of coordinating services and improvement activities

6. Supporting capital and new program requests and helping coordinate them with clinical units and other CSS

7. Maintaining the succession plan for the CSS

8. Arranging the resolution of inter- and intra-professional work requirements

9. Maintaining the agenda for contract renewal or restructuring of the relationship between the CSS and the HCO

The duty of contract renewal recognizes that there are alternative opportunities to provide many CSS. Even fully employed CSS should be reviewed periodically, and contractual relationships should have explicit revision or renewal dates. The HCO manager should monitor the array of alternatives and the improvement opportunities offered. Although the normal expectation would be for continuation of the relationship, the HCO's stakeholders are entitled to the best available arrangement. Review of alternatives may lead to a new supplier for the CSS; more commonly it identifies OFIs that can and should be addressed under the existing relationship.

SUGGESTED READINGS

Brunt, B. A. 2008. *Evidence-Based Competency Management for the Operating Room,* 2nd edition. Marblehead, MA: HCPro, Inc.

Hester, D. M. (ed.). 2008. *Ethics by Committee: A Textbook on Consultation, Organization, and Education for Hospital Ethics Committees.* New York: Rowman & Littlefield Publishers, Inc.

Papp, J. 2006. *Quality Management in the Imaging Sciences,* 3rd edition. St. Louis, MO: Mosby.

Reynolds, F. 2005. *Communication and Clinical Effectiveness in Rehabilitation.* Edinburgh, Scotland: Elsevier.

Chapter 9   In a Few Words . . .

Community health focuses on sustaining the health and productivity of all citizens. It includes extensive prevention, chronic disease management, all forms of acute and rehabilitative care, continuing care, and palliative care. It also emphasizes community safety, environmental protection, and health promotion. High-performing HCOs elect to pursue community health in addition to a narrower mission of excellent care. Community health has proven value and many advocates, but current (2010) HCO reimbursement does not reward a community health mission. HCOs that pursue community health use their management skills to do the following:

1. Analyze the full array of community health needs, forecasting demand for service, identifying current provider and stakeholder positions, developing OFIs for all levels of care, and advocating a community-wide response.
2. Establish a strategy to address specific needs through direct action, partnerships, and a broad-based community health advocacy group.
3. Operationalize the strategy through the advocacy group using the evidence-based and transformational management approaches.

Community health strategies use a unique set of strategic performance measures emphasizing population health and per capita healthcare cost. Under a community health mission, HCO senior managers must understand and teach concepts of both community health and evidence-based management. They often assist directly in governance roles for affiliated community health services and agencies.

Beyond Acute Care
to Community Health

Is This Your HCO?

Which of the following best describes your HCO?

HCO A: We strive to give each patient the best care. We focus on emergency wait times, screening for cancer and chronic disease, quick response with specialist referral and follow-up care, and having the equipment to supply the most up-to-date acute and rehab therapy. Specialist physicians dominate our medical staff. They expect us to support their practices, and we do.

HCO B: We want to keep our community healthy. Health insurance premiums and community disability and mortality measures are as important to us as Joint Commission quality scores. We participate in a community coalition to improve health. We run a hospice, and encourage all patients to complete advance directives. We give investment priority to primary care practices. Our specialists know that high tech capital requests will be funded only when the underlying science strongly supports improved patient outcomes.

This chapter describes HCO B: why some high-performing HCOs select it, what it means to operations, how to implement it, and how to measure it.

Community health focuses on sustaining all citizens at their highest possible level of functioning, for their individual happiness and for the collective benefit. It involves education, jobs, safety, and environment as well as healthcare. The healthcare component emphasizes comprehensive, integrated care for several levels of need: preventive, primary, acute, rehabilitative, continuing, and palliative. The healthcare component alone is substantially broader than the array of services most HCOs offer.

Several thousand communities have some sort of community health program. Several agencies promote the concept with examples and suggestions, including:

- American Hospital Association: Nova Awards (www.aha.org/ aha/news-center/awards/NOVA.html) and the Foster

McGaw Prize (www.aha.org/aha/news-center/awards/foster/index.html)

- Commission to Build a Healthier America (www.commissiononhealth.org/)
- Task Force on Community Preventive Services: *The Community Guide: What Works to Promote Health* (www.thecommunityguide.org/index.html)
- National Civic League (www.ncl.org/cs/services/healthy communities.html)
- The Kansas University Work Group for Community Health and Development (http://communityhealth.ku.edu/ctb/about_the_ctb.shtml)
- Healthy People Consortium (www.healthypeople.gov/Implementation/Consortium/default.htm)

WHAT DOES COMMUNITY HEALTH MEAN FOR HCOS?

For HCOs, the purpose of a community health mission is:

to use the HCO as a vehicle to improve community health.

The HCO's community health commitment can be in stages:

1. The commitment starts with excellence in patient care. Whatever the HCO's current role or roles, they should be approaching benchmark performance.
2. It extends to disease prevention, chronic disease management, continuing care, and end-of-life services. The community should have a full array of care services.
3. The next stage is a focus on keeping patients healthy. Health promotion, working with people who are not sick, pays off by reducing illness.

4. Finally, it links the HCO to other community agencies to reach high-risk markets effectively. The HCO can be a behind-the-scenes leader in many prevention and promotion activities.

In broad perspective, community health has solid empirical support. Residents of healthier communities live longer, have less disability, earn more money, and use less healthcare. In detail, however, moving to the ideal is challenging. Prevailing attitudes, organization structures, financing, and employment all must change.

The "community health" mission explicitly accepts the goal of a healthy community. The "excellence in care" mission assumes that the HCO's role is limited to the provision of selected parts of the care spectrum, usually those associated with acute treatment and rehabilitation. Examples of both appear in current mission statements of high-performing HCOs (see Exhibit 2.2). There are inherent conflicts of interest: if I am a cancer treatment specialist, prevention of cancer may reduce my future income. For an HCO, strong programs of community health may mean less hospital revenue, starting in places like oncology, cardiovascular care, and the neonatal intensive care unit. Community health is not financially supported under current payment mechanisms.

SHOULD OUR HCO MOVE TO COMMUNITY HEALTH?

When an HCO adopts a community health mission, it commits itself to address the structural problems of both financing and delivery of healthcare. Going beyond excellence in acute care will involve a substantial change in the HCO's role, but it represents a direction that will become increasingly important in the 21st century. Among other advantages, resources contributed to community health are included in the IRS Form 990 Schedule H Community Benefit calculations. In the future, excellent HCOs will adopt the community health mission, because it creates better communities and because the payment disincentives will be removed.

The decision should be supported by a strong foundation in acute care operations and financial performance and a plan to protect loyal associates whose income could be at risk. With that foundation, it's a really good idea. The healthier community that results will also be a richer community. The HCO will be positioned for success over the next several decades.

HOW DOES AN HCO PROMOTE COMMUNITY HEALTH?

The functions required to implement a community health mission are shown in Exhibit 9.1. They are framed in a way that allows a traditional HCO to move stepwise into community health—expanding via individual services and levels—or by developing a comprehensive response. The functions are applicable to *each* of the levels of care (prevention, primary, acute, rehab, home, continuing, and palliative) and to health promotion, as well as to *all* of those levels. The remaining questions in this chapter address implementation of the Exhibit 9.1 functions.

WHAT IS THE COMMUNITY HEALTH NEEDS ASSESSMENT?

A community health needs assessment:

1. identifies the community's health risks and potential risk reduction programs,
2. provides quantitative forecasts for specific services at each level of prevention and care using the epidemiologic planning model,
3. identifies current providers for each level of prevention and care,

Exhibit 9.1 Functions in Implementing a Community Health Mission

Function	Examples
Understanding and promoting community health	Working with health department and others to identify important local health issues
(a) Forecasting need and demand	Forecasting the demand and supply for specific services such as nursing home care
(b) Identifying intervention opportunities	
(c) Identifying stakeholder positions	Meeting with community groups to discuss needs and roles
(d) Advocacy and promotion of health behavior	Promoting smoking cessation, exercise programs, and reproductive health
Establishing a community health strategy	Building consensus around implications of expanded mission
(a) Community advocacy group	Developing expected outcomes, financial forecasts, and revised physician-need forecasts
(b) Mission	Analyzing alternative ownership and business models
(c) Performance measures	
(d) Financing	
(e) Market, competitive, and collaborative opportunities	

Exhibit 9.1 Continued

Function	Examples
Operationalizing community health	Implementing a strategic measures set and a business plan for a specific service such as a hospice or a home care program
(a) Service operations: Patient recruitment. Care planning. Staffing. Training. Budget and Finance. Continuous improvement.	Publicizing community health measures, benchmarks, and best practices
(b) Building an integrated network	Promoting consensus around realistic community health goals
(i) Promoting community health opportunities	
(ii) Establishing collaboration with existing units	
Improving performance	Conducting ongoing review of community health performance
(a) Identifying community health opportunities for improvement	Promoting achievements of advocacy group
(b) Developing collaborative approaches	Celebrating goals attained
(c) Building local understanding and contribution	Lobbying for changes in regulation and reimbursement
(d) Strengthening public commitment	

4. establishes OFIs that can be used to identify and prioritize a community health strategy, and

5. serves as the foundation for a program to educate stakeholders and promote interest in improvement.

Specific risks or conditions can be grouped in various ways to facilitate planning decisions. The full array of community health services is surprisingly large and diverse. Prevention and health maintenance services are available for many different population subgroups. Exhibit 9.2 shows groupings according to the level of prevention, the populations served, and the programs or organizations providing service. These groupings are important in designing responses.

1. The level of prevention is often key to the cost effectiveness and an important factor in prioritizing opportunities. Primary prevention is usually the most cost effective. Secondary prevention is much more problematic. Screening for existing disease has been a popular hospital activity, but its cost effectiveness depends upon minimizing false positives, usually by targeting high-risk groups. Tertiary prevention can be cost effective when it substantially reduces disability and hospital readmissions.
   The Centers for Disease Control and Prevention (CDC) Task Force on Community Preventive Services, www.thecommunityguide.org/index.html, categorizes over 200 preventive interventions as "Recommended," "Insufficient Evidence," or "Not Recommended."

2. The population served allows focused promotion and service, such as in high school–based programs for adolescents and medical home programs for chronic disease populations. The ability to focus both the marketing and care delivery is a major factor in reducing waste.

Exhibit 9.2 Disease and Prevention Forecasts Grouped by Prevention Level, Population, and Service Program

Prevention Level	Examples of Risks	Examples of Prevention Activity
Primary—Maintenance of health	Obesity, smoking, and substance abuse Environmental hazards	Dietary and exercise management "Child proofing" Smoking cessation Lead and asbestos removal Alcohol use laws
Primary—Prevention of specific disease	Infectious diseases Trauma Prematurity and birth defects Ischemic heart disease Stroke	Immunization, infection control Seat belts, helmets, alcohol management, domestic violence prevention Prenatal care Aspirin, anti-coagulants
Secondary—Early stage identification and elimination of disease	Cancer Diabetes Cardiovascular disease Developmental defects	Screening and early treatment Screening and dietary management Drug and lifestyle management Remedial child care
Tertiary—Reduction of the impact of chronic disease	Post-acute cardiovascular or stroke care, arthritis, trauma	Drug and lifestyle management Rehabilitation Home care and telemedicine

Continued

Exhibit 9.2 Continued

Population at Risk	Examples of Risks	Examples of Prevention Activity
High school students	Safe driving, health maintenance, substance abuse, sexual and reproductive activity	Classroom education, driver training, alcohol law enforcement, counseling services
Young families	Family planning, child safety, domestic abuse, health maintenance, disease screening	Maternal and reproductive health services, counseling, exercise programs, well baby services
Elderly	Functional losses, chronic disease, terminal illness	Home safety, rehabilitation programs, disease management, palliative care

Service Program	Examples of Risks	Examples of Prevention Site
Primary care	Acute disease, chronic disease, early detection, maternal and child health management	Medical homes, primary care offices, federally qualified health centers, industrial and school clinics, retail stores
Post-acute recovery	Post-operative rehabilitation	Hospital, rehabilitation center, nursing home
Continuing care	Diminished functional status, terminal illness	Home care program, nursing home, hospice

3. The service required is useful in identifying potential collaborators. Existing organizations can contribute important specialized knowledge and market contacts, making collaboration the strategy of choice in designing responses.

In addition to their role in planning, quantitative forecasts are used to set goals and evaluate results. Success is measured by reduction in incidence and prevalence. The Center for Health Care Strategies, www.chcsroi.org/Welcome.aspx, a group dedicated to improving the health of the chronically ill and otherwise disadvantaged people, offers a web-based return-on-investment model that allows comparison of alternative strategies.

HOW DOES THE NEEDS ASSESSMENT RELATE TO CURRENT PROVIDERS?

Few community health needs are totally ignored. Much more commonly, some existing organization is offering service, but the service falls short of need and benchmark. The inventory must include deliberate efforts to ensure that service meets standards for quality, effectiveness, patient satisfaction, and efficiency. Special attention is often necessary for disadvantaged populations. Care is often underfunded. Federally qualified health centers (FQHCs) and FQHC "look alikes" can be useful partners (see www.cms.hhs.gov/center/fqhc.asp). A Walmart business approach—careful program design, selective location, and continuous improvement of cost per case—is essential. This approach goes beyond efficiency. It continuously tests customer satisfaction against economy, seeking to eliminate all costs not essential to sustaining market share. It is substantially different from approaches to acute care, which has much richer financial support.

A substantial consensus on how to implement cost effective programs is now available on many elements of community health. The National Guideline Clearinghouse, www.guide-lines.gov, contains primary care guidelines for specific risks and age categories and disease-specific guidelines for home and end-of-life care. The Centers for Medicare & Medicaid Services MDS 3.0 program addresses issues that can identify opportunities to manage continuing care (www.cms.hhs.gov/Nursing-HomeQualityInits/25_NHQIMDS30.asp#).

The inventory might best be done by a collaborative community program that includes the organizations currently providing care as well as current and potential clients and payers. Forming a collaborative program is an important step in building stakeholder support and limiting special interest reactions.

WHAT'S THE COMMUNITY APPROACH TO COMMUNITY HEALTH?

Successful comprehensive community health strategies use a general community advocacy group to create a leadership structure. A community-oriented group is designed to bring together diverse interests and viewpoints. It usually begins with informal visits between individuals, expands to discussion sessions, and in many communities evolves to a formally appointed "commission" or "board" with a regular agenda and established relationships with major stakeholders. The initial discussions of stakeholder positions undertaken as part of the needs assessment provide the starting points. The needs assessment provides the focus.

Many communities already have advocacy groups. (See the web sources at the start of the chapter.) Once formed, the advocacy group builds consensus on strategy. It assumes independent authority and elects its leadership. It facilitates contracts between various stakeholders to implement the strategy.

HOW CAN AN HCO STIMULATE A COMMUNITY APPROACH?

Building collaboration between customer and provider stakeholders is frequently the key to community health success. A large HCO controls substantial market share, which can influence selected stakeholders, including competing HCOs. The list of potential collaborators is long. In most communities it includes:

- Government agencies in public health, welfare, education, environment, and justice. These agencies are frequently in touch with high-risk and disadvantaged populations.
- Employers. Many have a financial stake in success through reduced insurance premiums.
- Faith-based organizations. These organizations are a source of volunteers and can be effective at marketing community health programs.
- Civic and cultural organizations like United Way, homeless shelters, and YMCA.
- Other HCOs, including competitors in acute care and potential competitors in other levels of care, under both for-profit and not-for-profit organization. (There are potential anti-trust implications in any action taken directly with competitors. Although enforcement in comprehensive community care would be unusual, legal counsel is appropriate.)

Extensive listening is the foundation of collaborative activity. Community-oriented HCOs pursue an ongoing listening and relationship-building strategy that has several elements:

1. Routine surveillance of public information and reports
2. Personal contacts with leadership of important organizations

3. Monitoring of consumer interests through focus groups and surveys

4. Assisting groups with specific health interests with in-kind support, such as meeting space and computer linkage and funding

5. Establishing and maintaining contractual relationships. Hospitals have ongoing referral relationships with primary care physicians, nursing homes, rehabilitation services, home care services, and hospices. These relationships can be the foundation for expanded and improved activities and can include substantial HCO capital and operating investment.

6. Service on agency boards and committees by HCO managers and trustees and recognition in HCO activities. HCO associates are often willing to volunteer services to other community health organizations. Their knowledge of transformational and evidence-based management can be a valuable contribution. Similarly, leadership from other community health services can enrich HCO governance, planning, and improvement activities.

An HCO with a community health mission promotes general understanding. A communications plan for a community would include:

1. Identification of services and their importance

2. A summary of the needs assessment, promoted through a collaborative network including local media

3. Efforts to reach specific stakeholder interests through:
   — reports, factual summaries, and reference materials;
   — speakers' bureaus and planned communication to customer stakeholder segments; and
   — advertising and other promotion to increase customer awareness of individual services

4. Efforts to reach provider stakeholders with reliable information about demand, need, existing programs, and proposed programs

Competing HCOs can also be influenced by a well-designed strategy. They can be drawn into joint ventures or encouraged by market pressures to expand or improve services. A large HCO controls a substantial market share that it can direct to selected providers based on quality and cooperation.

The actions of HCOs are important reinforcement for community health concepts. High-performing HCOs do not allow smoking on site. Emphasis on patient safety is extended to the safety of their associates and guests. They provide and promote cost effective prevention for patients and families. They provide exercise opportunities, healthy meals, and counseling to their associates. They explicitly recognize patient autonomy and encourage the use of advance directives and designated patient advocates. They tailor their benefit programs to promote prevention and meet important health needs. These actions have both real and symbolic value.

WHAT DOES A MATURE COMMUNITY HEALTH PROGRAM LOOK LIKE?

Exhibit 9.3 describes the goals of a 15-year-old comprehensive community health program, Buffalo County Community Partners, located in Kearney, Nebraska. The program is notable for its quantitative measurement, "targets," and deliberate goal-setting. The goals are established by the governing board, which is drawn from a broad spectrum of the county. Trends are posted regularly from a variety of sources. The 2010 goals are Buffalo County's second set. The website indicates that only half the 15 goals set in 1996 were fully achieved, though some progress was made on almost all. The 2010 goal set includes several from the earlier list,

Exhibit 9.3 Goals of a Comprehensive Community Health Program

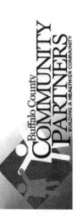

The vision of the Buffalo County Community Partners is that everyone from all corners of Buffalo County work together to improve the quality of life of those who live in and work in this community

BCCP Goals	Description	Results			Target
		2000	2003	2007	
Youth Who Smoke Regularly	. . . The last ten year focus has been on reducing secondhand smoke. Today they celebrate the new clean indoor air act . . .	24.8%	15.1%	11 %	12 %
Youth Marijuana Use	. . . county-wide strategic plan to reduce binge drinking, drinking and driving, and underage drinking.	14.2%	13.3%	10 %	5 %
Youth Binge Drinking		38 %	32.6%	23.2%	22.5%
Youth with Thoughts of Suicide	. . . strategy to increase mental health services in rural areas	15.3%	14 %	14 %	5 %
Health and Spirituality	To increase awareness of spirituality's effect on health and healing		79 %	86 %	Increase
Reducing Obesity (Overweight Adults)	To reduce obesity and overweight by increasing positive health behaviors relative to active living and nutrition	54 %	55 %	62 %	30 %
Smoke Free	To increase the percent of smoke free restaurants and businesses	100 %	47 %	77 %	100 %

Continued

Exhibit 9.3 Continued

BCCP Goals	Description	Results			Target
		2000	2003	2007	
Access to Health Care	To provide 100% access to health care for residents in Buffalo County	39 %*		42.9%**	0%
Safety: Seat Belt Use	To increase seat belt use to 80% of Buffalo County youth actively using their seat belts	76 %	79%	81 %	80%
Fall Prevention in Older Adults	To reduce falls in older adults (60+ year olds admitted to Good Samaritan Hospital)		42/1,000	31/1,000	Decrease
Lead	To decrease the percent of children exposed to lead	6.2%*		5.2%	0%
Affordable Housing	To increase the number of affordable housing units				
Transportation	Expand affordable public transportation services		55,280***	90,440	
Infant Mortality	To reduce infant mortality and post neonatal infant mortality	8.1/1,000	4.6/1,000	2.8/1,000	4.5/1,000

* Data for 1997
** Data for 2005
*** Data for 2001

SOURCE: Reprinted with permission from *2008 Report to the Community*. Buffalo County Community Partners, Kearney, NE.

but the board has regrouped them into broader market-oriented categories (www.bcchp.org/html/grants/2010actionplan.pdf).

HOW CAN COMMUNITY HEALTH PROGRAMS BE PROMOTED?

The final step in a community health strategy is the systematic use of the existing marketplace to expand the total use of appropriate services. This includes assisting existing organizations to improve and using collaborative opportunities to increase market penetration. Deliberate promotion, "social marketing," is essential for many community health activities. Coalitions with specific interest groups are valuable and completely consistent with social marketing concepts. Many groups with targeted missions have attracted the people most interested in their mission, the core "ready-to-buy" market. They form an invaluable nucleus for promotion. The acute care services can encourage appropriate referral.

HOW CAN COMMUNITY HEALTH PERFORMANCE BE MEASURED AND IMPROVED?

Community health service teams should be measured like any other healthcare team, using the operational dimensions of demand, cost, worker satisfaction, efficiency, quality, and customer satisfaction. Examples are shown in Exhibit 9.4. The teams conduct continuous improvement activities like all other teams.

In addition, individual community health programs are measured strategically in terms of their cost per case and cost per capita, as shown in Exhibit 9.5. These measures are used by the community advocacy group to identify strategic goals. The CDC's Task Force on Community Preventive Services has documented its measures and the evaluative process

Exhibit 9.4 Examples of Operational Measures for Community Health Programs

(*Note*: All programs will measure associate satisfaction and client satisfaction by survey. Program accounting records will measure resource consumption and counts of volumes, scheduling delays, and percent of capacity used.)

Program	Need/Demand	Productivity	Quality and Effectiveness
Well baby care	Incidence from birth data and forecasts Demand from existing programs	Cost per service (e.g., cost of standard vaccine packages) Cost per visit Cost per infant	Percent immunized Incidence of preventable condition reported (e.g., infectious disease, trauma, violence) Incidence of manageable condition reported (e.g., hearing, visual, or functional limitation)
Asthma management	Incidence per prevalence from epidemiologic model or survey Demand from existing programs	Cost per visit Cost per patient-year Cost per capita	Incidence of asthma-related disability from surveys (http://www.cdc.gov/asthma/questions.htm) Clinical data on asthmatic pulmonary function (outcomes) Clinical data on asthmatic treatment (process)

Continued

Exhibit 9.4 Continued

(*Note:* All programs will measure associate satisfaction and client satisfaction by survey. Program accounting records will measure resource consumption and counts of volumes, scheduling delays, and percent of capacity used.)

Program	Need/Demand	Productivity	Quality and Effectiveness
Home care	Waiting lists or unmet demand	Cost per visit	Patient, family, and physician satisfaction
	Comparison to similar communities	Cost per patient-month	Adverse events
	Demand from existing programs	Cost per capita	CMS OASIS C measures
Hospice	Waiting lists or unmet demand	Cost per visit	Patient, family, and physician satisfaction
	Comparison to similar communities	Cost per patient-month	Hospice referrals as percent of total mortality or disease-specific mortality
	Demand from existing programs	Cost per capita	Hospice-specific quality measures*
			The Dartmouth Atlas of Health Care 2008 Tracking the Care of Patients with Severe Chronic Illness

*Kirby, E. G., M. J. Keeffe, and K. M. Nicols. 2007. "A Study of the Effects of Innovative and Efficient Practices on the Performance of Hospice Care Organizations." *Health Care Management Review* 32 (4): 352–59.

(www.thecommunityguide.org/about/methods-ajpm-developing
guide.pdf;www.thecommunityguide.org/library/ajpm355
_d.pdf).

HOW DOES COMMUNITY HEALTH AFFECT HCO FINANCE?

Community health is a major vehicle to control long-term costs
but a potential threat to HCO revenue. The balance between the
two must be maintained by governing board policies. The policies
that have proven effective for HCOs with an acute care tradition
are the following:

- Every service must be planned and operated in a way that
  pursues continuous improvement to minimize cost and
  maximize appropriate revenue.
- Capital investments and deficit coverage are viewed as
  community dividends or benefits and are funded at the dis-
  cretion of the HCO board using three broad criteria:
  1. All funded activities should have a potential benefit that
     reasonably exceeds the support required, even though
     the benefit may be difficult to measure.
  2. The HCO's total investment cannot exceed prudent
     levels indicated in the long-range financial plan. (See
     chapters 3 and 13.)
  3. Acute care needs that keep the community competitive
     with others must take priority, because they are the
     HCO's core mission.

These criteria force collective consideration of all needs
including community health, provide a cost-benefit criterion for
prioritizing opportunities, and protect long-term stability. To protect the acute care activities, many high-performing HCOs set an
upper limit to investment in underfunded services. A few, such as

Exhibit 9.5 Community Health Strategic Scorecard

Dimension	Community Health Examples
Strategic measures of community health	Measures from government health statistics, such as: —mortality, by cause, with emphasis on preventable death; —natality, with emphasis on neonatal mortality, prematurity, and limitation; and —infectious disease rates. Measures from Medicare and Medicaid, such as: —per capita hospitalizations by diagnostic group, —incidence of chronic disease, —cost of hospitalization, and —cost of medical care in last two years of life. Measures from government agencies, such as: —domestic violence, —alcohol-related events, and —health and immunization of school children. Measures from community surveys, such as: —health insurance premiums; —health insurance coverage; —preventable emergency care; —pre-morbid and treatable conditions, including obesity, hypertension, depression; and —unfilled demand for health services.
Financial performance	Financial structure of advocacy group Grants and gifts for community health received by advocacy group and member organizations Financial performance of independent, affiliated, and wholly owned organizations supporting community health
Operations of care-giving units	Summary of OFIs from operations at each level of community health, drawn from their operational measures
Market performance and stakeholder satisfaction	Measures of access for disadvantaged groups Measures of cultural competence in healthcare Customer and provider stakeholder satisfaction

SSM Health Care and Catholic Health Initiatives, mandate a minimum as well.

WHAT ARE THE ANSWERS TO FAQS ABOUT COMMUNITY HEALTH?

As stakeholders contemplate the community health mission, several specific and practical questions are likely to arise, and the HCO spokespersons should be prepared to discuss them:

- Capital financial implications—how will the trade-off of community health and acute care be managed?
    1. Capital decisions for the HCO will continue to be made by its governing board in the overall interests of the community, recognizing both the importance of existing relationships and the HCO's unique role in acute care.
    2. The board intends to keep our community competitive with others in acute care. In all levels of care, the board will support investments that are scientifically sound, efficient in settings like ours, and generally accepted by health insurers.
    3. Our sound financial position allows us to do this, and the board is committed to maintaining that soundness.

    This answer places the question in context, clarifies the criteria, and states the philosophic position. It ensures that acute care will not be neglected.

- Provider income implications—how will these be managed? The answer:
    1. Reiterates the commitment to acute care needs from the first answer, pointing out the relevant specific opportunities that have been funded recently and noting that the HCO has in fact remained competitive.

2. Reiterates the HCO's commitment to using its medical staff planning function so that every physician has an opportunity to earn a competitive income by keeping the supply of high tech specialists in balance with clinically justified demand.

- Justice—"Should our HCO serve the needy or the insured, paying customer?" The answer notes:
    1. The HCO's not-for-profit status is justified in part by its contribution to addressing society's more general problems.
    2. The HCO will serve broader goals only to the extent external funding permits. That often means a specific limit on the funding to be transferred to uncompensated care.
- Faith-based restrictions on medical care—the expanded mission raises several potential areas of ethical conflict in addition to those inherent in acute care, such as reproductive health services and management of death.
    1. The non-religious not-for-profit HCO's position emphasizes patient autonomy—the right of each individual to choose his or her care for any reason, including reasons of faith.
    2. Religious HCOs have the right not to provide any treatment or service inconsistent with their faith.
    3. Both make an effort to avoid offending those who hold strong convictions.
    4. Potentially disturbing positions are implemented by carefully targeted promotion, location, corporate separation, and similar devices designed to isolate those desiring the service from those who find it offensive.

To be convincing, the HCO's answers to these questions must be backed by a record of trust and success. The record of leading hospitals shows that stakeholder reservations reflected in the questions can be overcome.

SUGGESTED READING

Commonwealth Fund. 2008. *The Path to a High Performance U.S. Health System: A 2020 Vision and the Policies to Pave the Way.* [Online information; retrieved 9/28/10.] www.commonwealthfund.org/Content/Publications/Fund-Reports/2009/Feb/The-Path-to-a-High-Performance-US-Health-System.aspx?page=all.

Fonseca-Becker, F., and A. L. Boore. 2008. *Community Health Care's O-Process for Evaluation.* New York: Springer.

National Center for Quality Assurance. 2008. *Standards and Guidelines for Physician Practice Connections—Patient-Centered Medical Home (PPC-PCMH).* Washington, D.C.: NCQA.

Office of Disease Prevention and Health Promotion, U.S. Department of Health and Human Services. *Healthy People 2020.* [Online information; retrieved 9/28/10.] http://www.healthypeople.gov/HP2020/.

Chapter 10   In a Few Words . . .

Knowledge management (KM) has become a core logistic support activity, providing the communication essential for care; defining, acquiring, and maintaining performance measures; and supporting learning activities. "Backstage" KM includes all forms of communication: the networks of voice, computer, and Internet used daily by associates and patients; the "data warehouse," an accessible archive of local data; and organized Internet access to useful external sources. KM protects data and the systems themselves and continuously improves its services. "Onstage," the benefits of KM come only through its customers—the clinical and other service units of the organization. In addition to supplying information, KM must interpret it and teach its applications. The KM planning committee is deeply involved in goal-setting, including goals for outside contractors. Its insights allow KM to generate revenue for its own expansion, finding areas where KM investment can easily be converted to performance improvement.

Knowledge Management

Is This Your HCO?

Ever since you hired the current chief information officer (CIO) (or signed the current contractor), the "backstage" KM stuff has disappeared from view. Hardware and software work. Reports come out on time, and the data in them are not challenged. The "roll-out" to the EMR is moving reasonably smoothly, after some first-round glitches. There's a sense that "we're finished with knowledge management." The KM planning committee is looked on as a dead-end job.

The frontier at this point is application: better measures and benchmarking (see "Specification and Adjustment"), better knowledge support in training programs and process improvement teams (PITs) (see "Turn Data to Knowledge"), and extended use of statistical process control (see "Random Variation"). The return is in actual performance: falling rates of unexpected events, quality and cost measures pushing close to benchmark, and PITs that uncover breakthrough process gains (see "Where Do We Get the Money"). The way to get there is encouragement by the Performance Improvement Council (PIC) and senior management, celebration, and collaborations that allow your HCO to copy best practice from others.

What to Do Next?

Three KM issues can threaten a program to reach excellence if they are mishandled.

Your coach points out that in each of these, the senior management team needs to implement the topics discussed in the chapter's nine questions.

1. The "backstage" isn't meeting competitive standards. Breakdowns, delays, and problems in the communications networks are so rare today that poor service is simply unacceptable. If performance does not promptly improve on the functions shown in Exhibit 10.1, the knowledge management leadership or the outside contractor must be replaced.

2. Associates are not convinced of the reliability of measures. When an operating team or a PIT looks at performance, the question should be "How do we reach benchmark?" not "There's something wrong with the measures" or "The measures are unfair." See the questions on reliability, specification, and random variation. Associate education and understanding ("Turning Data to Knowledge") are important. The strongest justifications for any measure are:

    a. other HCOs are using it and making benchmark, and
    b. it has been endorsed by national agencies such as National Quality Forum.

3. KM is underfinanced. KM, like all the logistic support services, should be viewed as an investment, rather than simply a cost. It's money you spend to get a return. The return comes in improved strategic performance, including net profit. The key goal-setting question for these units is not "How much are we spending?" It's "What is the evidence that a change in spending will translate to improved overall performance?" It's a harder question to answer, but the last

five questions in the chapter (turning data to knowledge, measuring KM performance, improving KM services, allocating funds, and using outside contractors)
all address the answer.

Knowledge management (KM) has become a major logistic support service that rivals human resources management and
boundary-spanning activities as a critical factor in HCO success.
KM services have an "onstage" duty to work continuously with
all other HCO units to improve the use of information and a
"backstage" duty to run a large, growing, and complex information utility. This chapter describes what KM must do to help
other units achieve high performance, emphasizing the "onstage"
interactions and leaving the "backstage" details to KM professionals.

The purpose of KM is:

**to translate the HCO's complete knowledge resource to
improvement of its strategic performance.**

The complete knowledge resource has four essential parts:

1. The knowledge, accumulated from many sources, that is in
   each associate's head.
2. The current communications driving the associates' agendas and recording their accomplishments.
3. The "data warehouse" of local information—protocols,
   processes, policies, performance data, proposals, and
   forecasts—that is part of the HCO's intranet.
4. The library of books and journals now increasingly on the
   Internet.

The knowledge resource must be supplied subject to the privacy rights of individuals, and it must be protected against distortion, loss, or misuse.

The "backstage" activities are expensive. Their cost must be supported by effective work processes in clinical, logistic, and strategic activities. The "onstage" role of KM facilitates the improvements that generate a return on the KM investment.

KM is inescapably tied to the electronic medical record (EMR). Most excellent HCOs are moving rapidly to implement the EMR, but it should be understood as a "backstage" improvement. The benefits of the EMR come from "onstage" application to processes that improve performance. Achieving them must involve all HCO units, not simply clinical ones.

WHAT ARE THE "BACKSTAGE" KM DUTIES?

KM must complete the five functions shown in Exhibit 10.1. These functions deliver information to end users at high standards of accuracy, comprehensiveness, confidentiality, and reliability. KM is an information utility that achieves reliability with redundancy.

HCOs require many special-purpose software sets, ranging from the EMR to the enterprise accounting system. KM must ensure that these software packages are integrated, use consistent definitions and standards, and provide appropriate security. KM manages the software licenses, including negotiating prices.

KM manages many hazards that may result in failure, distortion, and loss. The normal protections are individual identification systems and access limitation, physical protection of sites, duplication of records and systems, separate geographic locations of originals and duplicates, selection of personnel, and antivirus software. KM must have a formal plan for maintaining protection and confidentiality and a recovery plan for

Exhibit 10.1 Functions of Knowledge Management Services

Function	Content
Ensure the reliability and validity of data	Defines measures and terminology
	Supports accurate, complete data input
	Applies appropriate specification and adjustment
	Estimates reliability of data
Maintain data communications for daily operations	Operates a 24/7 electronic and voice communication utility
	Supports software used in clinical and business functions
	Integrates information from multiple applications
Support information retrieval for continuous improvement	Retrieves and integrates historical data, supports Web access for research, and provides comparative data for management and clinical decisions
	Provides protocols, processes, training videos, and other materials supporting training programs
	Provides training in the use of automated systems and consulting service in information availability and interpretation
Ensure the appropriate use and security of data	Guards against loss, theft, and inappropriate application
Continuously improve knowledge management services	Establishes a prioritized agenda for progress
	Incorporates user views
	Commits a block of capital funds for several years
	Supports an annual review of specific projects

each of the perils. KM is responsible for maintaining this plan, including monitoring effectiveness and conducting periodic drills for specific disasters.

HOW DOES AN HCO ENSURE RELIABILITY OF MEASURES?

In a world that relies on measurement, the accuracy of the measures becomes critical. Four steps are necessary to minimize measurement errors: (1) standard definitions, (2) consistent application, (3) statistical specification and adjustment, and (4) estimation of residual variation and confidence limits. In excellent HCOs, KM supports an interdisciplinary committee that oversees the definitions, standardization, specification, adjustment, and interpretation of measures. Sharp HealthCare, a 2008 Malcolm Baldrige National Quality Award (MBNQA) recipient, identifies the following criteria for measures:

- Reference in evidence-based literature
- Use by regulatory and public reports
- Availability of competitor data
- Use by other MBNQA recipients
- Availability of benchmarks in healthcare and beyond

The committee's decisions are incorporated into educational programs and software to ensure consistent application. The committee audits use of standard definitions on its own or through internal audit mechanisms.

Standard definitions must be rigorously applied to each transaction. Commercial software is available for most information capture operations. It is designed for accurate entry and user convenience, includes extensive edits and audits, and facilitates prompt retrieval and linkage across multiple data sources.

WHAT DO SPECIFICATION AND ADJUSTMENT MEAN?

Some random variation always remains when human caregivers treat human patients. As the data are aggregated over time and work sites, questions of comparability arise: How can population A be made more comparable to population B? Specification and adjustment allow apples-to-apples comparison; they are critical in many clinical measures and valuable in many forecasts and marketing analyses. Specification defines more homogeneous subpopulations within a larger, more heterogeneous population. It is necessary whenever parts of the total population have different responses to the measure in question, and the parts vary for reasons outside the organization's control. For example, hip-replacement recovery rates can be specified by age and the degree of loss of function prior to surgery. Acute myocardial infarction survival can be specified by age, gender, and the presence of other disease. All these factors are arguably outside the treatment teams' control. (The process of specification is analogous to "segmentation" in marketing and is discussed further in Chapter 15.)

Adjustment recalculates the whole population rate from the specific rates, standardizing to the characteristics of a single population. For example, local mortality rates are adjusted to the age and sex of the U.S. population as a whole. The age-adjusted rate for each state is the mortality rate it would have if its population had the same age distribution as the nation's. The 50 states can then be compared and ranked. Many nationally defined clinical measures are adjusted for multiple factors to remove characteristics beyond the caregivers' control and allow fair comparison to trend or benchmark. The possibility of an omitted variable remains, however. It should be raised as part of a root cause analysis: "Are there any other factors outside the unit's control that we should consider?"

SHOULD PERFORMANCE MEASURES ADDRESS RANDOM VARIATION?

Few performance measures are exact. Commonly used measures such as laboratory test values, cost per case, length of stay, percentage of patients "loyal," and percentage of patients surviving are all subject to random variation that can mislead users. Adjustment reduces, but never removes, random variation. Confidence limits estimate the probability that a specific difference is worth investigating. Investigating noise (W. Edwards Deming's "special causes," meaning factors that are unique and may not recur) is a waste of time; when a variation is significant (Deming's "common causes") an investigating team is likely to be able to find a cause for the difference. The "level of significance" is the probability that a cause can be found. "Significant at 95 percent" is a forecast that 19 times out of 20, a diligent team will find a potentially correctible cause.

The usual variability indicators are the standard deviation (used to compare two individual values) and the standard error (used to compare two samples with several individual values in each). Modern statistical process control software calculates both measures, shows trends and significance graphically, and automatically flags significant differences.

HOW DO HCO ASSOCIATES TURN DATA TO KNOWLEDGE?

The data warehouse and the Internet help associates retrieve information. Examples of important uses of information are shown in Exhibit 10.2. "Backstage," data management and modeling techniques allow KM workers to map the sources of the data and the calculations they need to forecast trends, analyze relationships, and model alternative approaches.

Exhibit 10.2 Common Uses of Information in High-Performing HCOs

Application	"Data Warehouse" Information	Internet Information
Reporting performance	Recent data relative to goals Graphs, statistical process control	
Identifying OFIs	"Drill down" to identify potential causes Local benchmarks and comparative performance	Journal articles, collaboratives, and comparative information
Setting goals	Local trends, benchmarks, and forecasts	External benchmarks and best practices
Supporting PITs	Analytic models, simulations, and forecasts	Books and journal articles, regulatory standards, recommended practices
Reviewing protocols	Reported variances from protocol "Drill down" of outcomes to show patient-specific groups Analytic models, simulations	National clearinghouses, commission reports, journal articles, books
Managing individual patients		Journal articles, guidelines, diagnostic software

"Onstage," KM works with other units to provide comprehensive training in using the reports for improvement. Much of the training is delivered just-in-time, as the need for understanding is encountered. For example, a PIT studying an admissions process decides that associates involved in patient registration need training in approaching patients and families, understanding confidentiality and elementary rules about guardianship, using the input screens, and learning the appropriate definitions. Most important, they need to know when they need help and where to get it. Human resources and the unit manager will provide most of this training, but KM will be involved at several steps:

1. A video describes the HCO's mission, vision, and values. A second might expand the HCO's policies regarding relations with patients and associates, dress, and compensation and benefits.
2. A training module teaches completion of electronic forms for data entry. The module can include a test with multiple scenarios testing the associate's understanding.
3. Guardianship, HIPAA, and advance directive materials are summarized on the company intranet and backed with specific procedures. A workshop makes associates more comfortable and effective with these sensitive issues.
4. Mastery of key rules is tested, using computerized test procedures.
5. A set of FAQs is supplemented by the associate's own notes.
6. Models of the operation help identify the performance improvement that justifies the investment.

Training for more complex tasks is accomplished similarly, by breaking the process into components and providing instruction or support on each component. Thus, very sophisticated systems can be built. For example, patient diagnosis is translated to ICD codes by clerical employees and coded to diagnosis-related groups (DRGs) or ambulatory patient classifications by programmed algorithms. The ICD coders have access to code lists with definitions and examples, interpretations of terminology, training in review of the record to catch diagnoses omitted by the physician (a review that can be automated in the EMR), and access to a knowledgeable nosologist or supervisor trained in clinical coding. They can specialize in a limited set of diseases. They also have the option of returning to the physician for further clarification. Finally, a blind test can be run to check intercoder consistency, and audits can be focused on the codes that result in the most errors.

The electronic training resources provide a system that documents mastery at Kirkpatrick level 3 (application, see Chapter 11), both confirming learning and building the associate's confidence.

HOW IS KM PERFORMANCE MEASURED?

Performance measures for KM should cover the full set of six dimensions shown in Exhibit 10.3. A large number of specific activity measures can be devised to supplement the list in Exhibit 10.3. The KM planning committee will have an important role in negotiating KM's annual goals.

HOW ARE KM SERVICES CONTINUOUSLY IMPROVED?

KM requires a sophisticated planning process for continuous improvement, such as the one shown in Exhibit 10.4, managed by a KM planning committee or steering committee. The charge to the KM planning committee includes the following:

- Participate in the development of the KM plan, resolve the strategic priorities, and recommend the plan to the governing board

Exhibit 10.3 Measures of KM Performance

Dimension	KM Function	Measure
Demand	Reliability and validity of data	New measure requests, response time
		"Hits" on data warehouse materials
		Counts of measures in place
	Data communications	System users
		System peak users
	Information retrieval	Counts of measures, benchmarks in use
		Counts of service requests
		Counts of trainees
	Appropriate use and security	Protection systems enabled
		Real and mock assaults managed
	KM planning and improvement	Projects managed
Costs and resources	All	Units and costs of resources
		Capital expenditure
		Machine capacity
Human resources	All	Associate satisfaction, retention, absenteeism, work loss days

Exhibit 10.3 Continued

Dimension	KM Function	Measure
Output and productivity	All	Counts of services completed
		Productivity measures divide cost incurred by counts of service completed
Quality	Reliability and validity of data	Counts of measures benchmarked
		Statistical tests of reliability, sensitivity
		Audit scores
	Data communication	Response delay
		Systems uptime
		Audit scores
		Unexpected events
	Information retrieval	Trainee mastery scores
	Appropriate use and security	Audit scores
		System attacks
		Consultant ratings
	KM planning and improvement	Projects on time
		Projects on budget
		Projects meeting original performance goals
Customer satisfaction	All	Customer surveys, interviews, complaints, unexpected events

Exhibit 10.4 Knowledge Management Planning Process

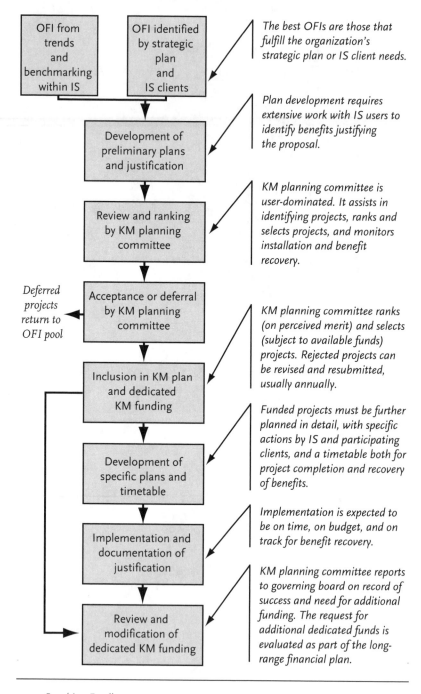

OFI from trends and benchmarking within IS	
OFI identified by strategic plan and IS clients	*The best OFIs are those that fulfill the organization's strategic plan or IS client needs.*
Development of preliminary plans and justification	*Plan development requires extensive work with IS users to identify benefits justifying the proposal.*
Review and ranking by KM planning committee	*KM planning committee is user-dominated. It assists in identifying projects, ranks and selects projects, and monitors installation and benefit recovery.*
Acceptance or deferral by KM planning committee	*KM planning committee ranks (on perceived merit) and selects (subject to available funds) projects. Rejected projects can be revised and resubmitted, usually annually.*
Inclusion in KM plan and dedicated KM funding	*Funded projects must be further planned in detail, with specific actions by IS and participating clients, and a timetable both for project completion and recovery of benefits.*
Development of specific plans and timetable	
Implementation and documentation of justification	*Implementation is expected to be on time, on budget, and on track for benefit recovery.*
Review and modification of dedicated KM funding	*KM planning committee reports to governing board on record of success and need for additional funding. The request for additional dedicated funds is evaluated as part of the long-range financial plan.*

Deferred projects return to OFI pool

- Rank KM investment opportunities and recommend a rank-ordered list of proposals to the governing board
- Assist KM clients in identifying and meeting KM opportunities
- Support the definitions and standards committee
- Monitor performance of the division, and suggest possible improvements

The KM planning committee routinely includes key personnel from major departments, particularly finance, internal consulting, medicine, nursing, and clinical support services. The CIO is always a member and may chair the committee. Members of the governing board may serve on the committee. The team uses a variety of task forces and subcommittees, expanding participation in component activities but using its authority to coordinate.

The processes the committee manages should have several important characteristics:

- They are built around explicit collaboration with application units, because KM cannot itself control the results. Most proposals are four-part:

    1. A KM change (new hardware, software, or information capability) will be installed in some HCO activity other than KM.
    2. The installation will support improved work processes.
    3. The improved work processes will improve operational measures.
    4. Improved operations will create improvements in HCO strategic measures. (For example, software to improve patient scheduling in outpatient offices will increase the

number of patients who can be seen. If marketing and other parts of the primary care service line are effective, outpatients seen and correctly treated will increase. As outpatient visits increase, HCO revenue and profit will increase.)

- They establish project teams with detailed goals, analogous to facility construction projects. (For the outpatient improvement project, the PIT must include primary care, nursing, marketing, and KM. It is likely to work through a battery of subteams establishing the software vendor, pilot tests, an installation timetable, revised patient management protocols, and an associate training plan. The PIT will have associates or contractors accountable for progress and operational improvement.)
- The project teams are monitored by the KM planning committee. (The several project teams will need the planning committee as a coordinating body.)
- Funding is established on a multi-year basis, usually by allocating a portion of the total funds available for new programs and capital to KM projects. (The amounts, the benefits, and the timetables will be built into the long-range financial plan and other planning activities.)
- The governing board's review focuses on two questions, "What are the strategic improvements that justify the investment?" and "How closely do the documented successes from installed projects track the benefits expected?" (The board's questions put a premium on KM performance and enforce continuous improvement of internal operations.)

WHERE DO WE GET THE MONEY FOR KM?

KM is expensive. All of these steps—capital for KM equipment, planning project implementation teams, subcommittees and task forces removing roadblocks—take time and money. Many HCOs struggle to find adequate funding. The question is a variation on the perennial "How can I drain the swamp when I'm surrounded by alligators?" The record of excellent HCOs shows that this question has a two-part answer.

Part one is the deliberate search for easy gains, "low-hanging fruit." The documented experience has shown that most HCOs have readily available KM improvements that pay off simultaneously in reduced wasted staff time, better quality, and lower costs. An important part of this dynamic is reduced clinical error. Under DRG payment, errors erode profit; fewer errors mean shorter stays, lower cost per case, and higher margins. If the initial KM projects are well selected and well implemented, they will generate cash flow.

Part two is to assess cost budgets with great care. While resource consumption is important, the central management question regarding KM is not "How much are we spending?" but "What are we getting for the money?" and "How much *should* we spend?" It is possible to operate KM at an insufficient scale and not recognize it. The customers of KM may be satisfied with service. The cost may be below reported benchmarks. The critical test, which must be explored by the board finance committee, senior management, and the KM planning committee, is not whether current performance is acceptable, but whether an additional investment would gain important returns. One way to approach this is to commission a periodic audit by an outside expert, who can compare service as well as cost and identify the technological opportunities. In addition, the audit team can evaluate all the KM activities in light of achievements of others.

HOW CAN KM USE OUTSIDE CONTRACTORS AND VENDORS?

Support available from outside contractors can include integrated software, finance, consultation and planning, facilities management, and joint development ventures. Most HCOs use at least some outside support. The contractor must fulfill the same "onstage" and "backstage" roles as employed associates. The operational measures and progress toward benchmark evaluate either structure.

The KM planning committee remains in place. It has a major role in selecting and working with contractors. It negotiates the annual performance goals. Contractors have no incentive to limit the hospital's costs and usually will profit from an excessive program for improvement. Thus, even with a facilities management contract, the KM planning committee and hospital governance have the responsibility to require justification, select improvements, and pace the evolution of the information system.

Healthcare systems generally centralize much of KM. They standardize definitions to provide comparative and benchmarking data. They require complete standardization of accounting and internal auditing, which virtually mandates standard software. They can frequently negotiate volume discounts on hardware and software. Training, local planning, and some user support for clinical and other systems must remain decentralized, although teaching aids can be standardized and modern communication allows expert backup that was formerly obtainable only from consultants. The performance measures are critical, as they are in selecting outside vendors. Each hospital in the system is entitled to service and price as good as or better than it could achieve on its own. But each hospital is obligated to produce and implement a plan of KM improvement.

SUGGESTED READINGS

Glandon, G. L., D. H. Smaltz, and D. J. Slovensky. 2008. *Austin and Boxerman's Information Systems for Healthcare Management,* 7th edition. Chicago: AUPHA/Health Administration Press.

Green, M. A., and M. J. Bowie. 2007. *Essentials of Health Information Management: Principles and Practices.* Stamford, CT: Delmar Cengage Learning.

McWay, D. C. 2003. *Legal Aspects of Health Information Management.* Clifton Park, NY: Thomson/Delmar Learning.

Wager, K. A., F. W. Lee, and J. P. Glaser. 2009. *Health Care Information Systems: A Practical Approach for Health Care Management,* 2nd edition. San Francisco: Jossey-Bass.

Chapter 11   In a Few Words . . .

An HCO's associates, its human resource, constitute its most valuable and improvable asset. Their "loyalty" (commitment to the mission and willingness to recommend to others) and "learning" (ability to identify, design, and implement improvements) measure their worth. Human resources management (HRM) provides support to retain, recruit, train, develop, and compensate all associates. In high-performing HCOs, HRM:

- Plans workforce needs, including management succession.
- Recruits and selects highly motivated associates reflecting the community's cultural makeup.
- Trains associates and managers to implement the mission, vision, and values.
- Supports training in technical and professional skills.
- Provides counseling and development programs that encourage individual growth.
- Develops highly competitive compensation and incentive payment systems.
- Designs and implements highly responsive employment benefit plans.

Excellent HCOs invest more than twice average levels in HRM. HRM makes over 80 contact hours per full-time equivalent (FTE) per year, mostly in training and coaching. The return for the investment comes in retention of trained, motivated, knowledgeable associates who accomplish more, make fewer mistakes, and consistently "delight" patients and other customers.

Human Resources Management

Is This Your HCO?

Communicating the mission, vision, and values required a whole new approach to new employee orientation. HRM has emerged as important in countless process improvement teams (PITs). Every new process seems to need a new training program. Rounding raised a raft of employee concerns about pay, benefits, schedules, working conditions, and safety. Incentive pay went into place for all employed associates. HRM had to design and manage it. Overall, the result was major improvements in associate satisfaction, attendance, and retention.

"Are we there yet?"

Your coach says:

You're there if the measures of the human resource shown in Exhibit 11.3 are all at benchmark. Then the challenge becomes staying there. Some of the components that make the initial gains permanent are covered in some of the HRM questions in this chapter:

How Does HRM Support Transformational Management?
What's in the Workforce Plan?

What Can Be Done about Diversity and Cultural Competence?

How Are Leaders Developed?

What Is Service Recovery?

Can HRM Do Continuous Improvement?

What to Do Next?

Adequate nurse staffing is an opportunity for improvement (OFI) that just won't go away. Nurse satisfaction and retention are high, but finding enough people is a problem.

The answer has three main components, all of which depend on HRM:

1. Maintain the workforce plan, and a community recruitment program to go with it. Subsidize advancement on every step of the nursing career ladder. Assist schools with career opportunity programs. Assist college education with faculty support, field sites, and scholarships.
2. Maintain the environment and culture that nursing associates seek. (This includes transformational management, diversity, benefits, a safe and supportive workplace, and complaint management.)
3. Work continuously on moving tasks to lower skilled associates. This requires cooperation from clinical caregivers, but in a well-managed environment it is clearly in their interests. Training is the key. Using patient management and functional protocols (Chapter 5) opens the possibility of teaching less trained personnel and delegating components of care while keeping a safe, patient-sensitive environment.

The purpose of human resources management (HRM) is:

to increase the contribution of the human resource to the HCO's mission by designing and implementing appropriate policies and programs.

The HCO's human resource is its associates—employees, physicians, contract workers, and volunteers. Each associate joins the HCO in a voluntary exchange transaction seeking some combination of income, rewarding activity, society, and recognition. HRM works to optimize that exchange transaction.

WHAT IS THE NEW MODEL IN HRM?

Twenty-first century HRM is different from earlier HRM in three ways:

1. HRM is directly involved with sustaining the transformational culture throughout the HCO. The four characteristics that emerge from the literature as promoting that contribution are as follows:
   a. Group cohesiveness and effective teamwork, particularly the role of a responsive supervisor.
   b. Guaranteed individual rights.
   c. Some form of profit sharing or gain sharing.
   d. Job security and long-term employment.
   HRM works to ensure those characteristics for every job and all associates.
2. HRM is managed by measurement of the workforce. Data on associate satisfaction, training, retention, safety, and absenteeism are systematically mined for OFIs that push toward benchmark.

3. Training emerges as the new priority. Traditional HCOs provide 20 hours of training per FTE per year. Excellent ones provide 80 hours to more than 100 hours.

WHY DOES THE NEW MODEL PAY OFF?

The new model pays off because:

1. Fewer than 10 percent of associates leave each year. Over 90 percent remain. This means:
   a. The cost of recruiting and training new workers, equivalent to several months' pay, is vastly reduced.
   b. The investment in training has a much longer payoff. Most associates will remain with the HCO for more than five years.
2. Work teams are more stable, more knowledgeable, and more experienced.
3. Empowered, loyal associates, confident of themselves and their teams, handle their work more efficiently and more effectively.

HOW DOES HRM SUPPORT TRANSFORMATIONAL MANAGEMENT?

Transformational management—the concepts of empowerment, responsive listening, and service excellence—began to spread widely in the United States only after 1980. It represents a profound change in managerial behavior, essentially from "order giving" to "listening, responding, and encouraging." Much of the folklore of American industry runs counter to the realities of transformational supervision. HRM uses multiple educational approaches and media to reinforce basic notions: the role of responsive listening, the importance of clear instructions and appropriate work environments, the importance of fairness and candor, and the use of rewards rather than sanctions. Cases, role-playing, recordings, films, and individual counseling are helpful.

HRM trains managers to be responsive in applying the organization's policies on the protection of confidentiality, the promotion of diversity, and the elimination of sexual harassment and workplace hostility. HRM explains compensation and benefits, incentive programs, and policy application. Supervisors can guide associates to HRM's intranet on relevant procedures. When they are insufficient, HRM counselors assist. HRM also trains managers in running the PITs and other meetings essential to transformational decision making. HRM teaches how to make meetings start on time, end on time, have an agenda with appropriate supporting materials and minutes, and accomplish the agenda. HRM coaching can help chairs prepare effective agendas and minutes, make sure all participants are heard, keep to the topic and schedule, and promote consensus.

WHAT FUNCTIONS DOES HRM CONTRIBUTE TO HIGH PERFORMANCE?

The functions of HRM are shown in Exhibit 11.1. They are mostly "onstage," but each requires a substantial "backstage" capability. The questions that follow address the most critical issues in terms of general HCO needs and obligations—what HRM must do for the HCO to succeed.

Exhibit 11.1 Functions of Human Resources Management

Function	Description	Example
Workforce planning	Development of employment needs by job category	Forecast of RNs required and available by year
	Strategic responses in recruitment, downsizing, training, and compensation	Strategy for recruitment, retention, and workforce adjustment
Workforce development	Recruitment	Advertising, school visits
	Selection	Credentials review, interviewing
	Orientation	Review mission/vision/values, key workplace policies
	Training	Specific skill training and continuous improvement courses
	Diversity and cultural competence	Special programs for women and minorities

Exhibit 11.1 *Continued*

Function	Description	Example
Workforce maintenance	Services	Health promotion, child care, and social activities
		Counseling, grievance, and collective bargaining management
	Safety	Accident reduction programs and OSHA reports
	Records	Personnel records, including special competencies
		Satisfaction survey and analysis
	Reduction	Attrition management, retirement
Empowerment, transformation, and service excellence	Management education	Programs of human relations skills, continuous improvement skills, and meeting management skills
	Service recovery	Programs in service standards
		Training for service recovery

Continued

Exhibit 11.1 *Continued*

Function	Description	Example
Compensation and benefits management	Market surveys of compensation	RN pay scales, RN benefit selection, and benefit cost
	Payroll management	Compensation, incentives, absenteeism, and benefits-use records
	Benefits design and administration	Health insurance, retirement, and vacation benefit
Collective bargaining	Response to organizing drives, contract negotiation, and contract administration	Management of union collective bargaining contracts
Continuous improvement	Ongoing review of performance of the associate force	Identification of potential shortage situations and recruitment or retention difficulties
	Ongoing review of HRM activities	Continued improvement of workforce satisfaction, retention, and safety
	Identification of OFIs and establishment of improvement goals	Human resources department operational scorecard improvements

WHAT IS IN THE WORKFORCE PLAN?

The workforce plan is a subsection of the organization's strategic plan (see Chapter 14). It includes the following:

- Anticipated numbers of associates needed by skill category, major site, and department by year for three to five years in the future
- Schedule of adjustments through recruitment, retraining, attrition, and termination
- Succession plan for key managerial positions
- The medical staff plan (see Chapter 6)
- Wage and benefit cost forecasts
- Summary of HRM activities that will allow the plan to become reality

The workforce plan must be updated annually as part of the environmental assessment, along with other parts of the organization-wide strategic plan. A task force—including representatives from human resources, planning, finance, nursing, and medicine—guides the effort. The concerns of service lines and support units must be resolved. The revised plan is coordinated with the facilities plan and the long-range financial plan. It is recommended to the governing board through its planning committee.

The human resources department works closely with the employing departments to translate the plan to workforce adjustments and plans for individuals. Guidelines for the use of temporary labor (such as overtime, part-time, and contract labor) and compensation, incentive, and benefit design arise from the workforce plan.

The payoff from the plan is three-fold:

1. Recruitment strategies improve hiring of scarce professionals. Nursing, primary care, and several other clinical areas are likely shortage areas. Leading HCOs promote health careers beginning in kindergarten.

2. The succession plan encourages systematic preparation for departures and promotions, and builds bench strength.

3. Advance notice reduces the trauma involved in workforce adjustments and makes it possible to repay associate loyalty with job security.

HOW IS THE WORKFORCE MANAGED?

Building and maintaining the best possible workforce requires recruitment, selection, training, and managing diversity. Most of these functions are provided in close collaboration with the associates' work units.

Excellent HCOs are increasingly emphasizing cultural competence, making an effort to balance all levels of the workforce to the community population. They encourage self-screening by showing potential applicants the mission, vision, and values of the organization and the detailed job description. They use screening activities and background checks to further narrow the pool and often use structured interviews with the few remaining candidates. The final selection is made by the work team leader.

Search committees are frequently used for higher supervisory levels and medical staff leaders. HRM acts as staff for the search committee while ensuring that the recruitment protocol has been met. Internal promotion is often desirable for these positions. A succession plan identifies the candidates for promotion and prepares these candidates so that the HCO is protected against manager loss.

WHAT IS THE ROLE OF TRAINING?

Training is a major component of HRM activity and an important aspect of associates' work life. Training begins immediately upon hiring. It averages about 10 days per year for full-time employees, with managerial associates receiving above-average opportunities. The array of offerings in a large HCO includes:

- orientation;
- legally required information on safety, confidentiality, and civil rights;
- technical skills related to the specific job;
- continuous improvement and performance measurement;
- guest relations programs;
- work policy changes;
- retirement planning;
- outplacement assistance;
- benefits management;
- management of major organizational changes; and
- formal continuing education.

Operating units and healthcare professionals are frequently directly involved. An effort is made to make the educational programs participatory and applications-oriented. As noted in Chapter 2, all of these programs should be routinely evaluated at 3 Kirkpatrick levels (level 1 is recipient satisfaction, level 2 is content mastery, and level 3 is application). It is difficult to attribute actual performance improvement (Kirkpatrick 4) to specific training, but surveys, observation, and operating records can confirm that the training supports continuous improvement.

WHAT CAN BE DONE ABOUT DIVERSITY AND CULTURAL COMPETENCE?

Most leading HCOs strive to promote diversity in their workforce, but limited evidence suggests that women and minorities are still underrepresented in management. The more successful HCOs adapt job requirements to family needs and work to promote women in management. Increasing attention to the needs of female workers has clearly influenced the structure of employment benefits and the rules of the workplace.

Language, religion, culture, and unconventional views of illness and treatment can reduce patient compliance and satisfaction, and ultimately impair outcomes. The Joint Commission plans more specific cultural and linguistic standards in 2011. Leading HCOs measure cultural diversity, establish goals for service, and evaluate effectiveness of cultural and linguistic services. Cultural competence needs are met by training, coaches, ethics committees, and counselors. Linguistic services include multi-lingual/multi-cultural staff, trained medical interpreters, and qualified translators.

WHAT IS NEW IN THE BENEFIT PACKAGE?

Most HCOs provide employment benefits to their employees. What's new is cafeteria plans, which tailor offerings to employees' needs. Popular programs are allowed to grow, while others are curtailed. Charges are sometimes imposed to defray the costs, but some subsidization is usual. Workplace wellness and employee assistance programs have been shown to reduce absenteeism and health insurance costs. Child care also reduces absenteeism. The result is a complex program of services that requires a "backstage" management team.

HOW DOES AN HCO MAINTAIN A SAFE, COMFORTABLE WORKPLACE?

HRM is responsible for meeting the requirements of the Occupational Safety and Health Act—including submitting statistics to authorities—and for enforcing sexual harassment policies. The regulations in both of these areas recognize and reward careful prevention efforts.

Excellent HCOs keep work-related illness and injury low by constant attention to safety. Healthcare is not a safe industry. It lags behind the all-industry average and has not improved as much. Back injuries, needle sticks, and associate infections are preventable. Hazards such as radioactivity or anesthesia gases can be reduced.

Much of the direct control of hazards is the responsibility of the clinical engineering and facilities maintenance departments. Infection control, for example, is an important collaborative effort of housekeeping, plant engineering, nursing, and medicine. HRM is usually assigned the following functions:

- Monitoring and analyzing safety and complaint measures, benchmarks, federal and state regulations, and professional literature for HCO-wide OFIs.
- Maintaining material safety data sheets. These are profiles of hazardous substances with information on safe handling, which must be filed with the Occupational Safety and Health Administration and systematically distributed to associates who are exposed to the substances.
- Providing or assisting with training in and promotion of safe procedures.
- Negotiating contracts for workers' compensation insurance or, in the case of HCOs that self-insure, managing settlements.

DO EXCELLENT HCOS EVER HAVE LAYOFFS?

Changes in population, technology, competition, payment for care, and the economy can force any HCO to make substantial involuntary reductions in its workforce. Good practice pursues the following rules:

- Workforce planning is used to foresee reductions as far in advance as possible, allowing natural turnover and retraining to provide much of the reduction.
- Temporary and part-time workers are reduced first.
- Personnel in at-risk jobs are offered priority for retraining programs and new positions that arise.
- Early retirement programs are used to encourage older (and often more highly compensated) employees to leave voluntarily.
- Terminations are based on seniority or well-understood rules, judiciously applied.

Using this approach has allowed many HCOs to limit involuntary terminations to a level that does not seriously impair the attractiveness of the organization to others.

HOW ARE ASSOCIATE COMPLAINTS HANDLED?

Well-managed HCOs provide an authority independent of the normal accountability for employees who feel, for whatever reason, that their complaint or question has not been fully and fairly answered. The function of the counselor is to settle complaints fairly and quickly and to identify corrections that will prevent recurrence. Success depends on meeting worker needs before they develop into confrontations or serious dissatisfaction. Good grievance management begins with management training in responsive listening. When disagreements arise, good grievance administration documents, analyzes, and resolves the underlying situation. In the rare cases that go to arbitration or review, the HCO expects a favorable decision. The processes are appropriate in both union and non-union environments.

HOW ARE LEADERS DEVELOPED?

Managers have a critical role in transformational management; they must exhibit the behaviors required and provide much of the just-in-time education. Non-health companies report up to 80 hours of managerial training per manager per year. A growing number of leading healthcare systems are making similar investments. The topics focus on human relations and supervisory skills, facts about policies and procedures, managing PITs and collaborative activities, and mastery of tools for continuous improvement.

Skills to identify, evaluate, and implement improvement opportunities and to motivate associates are usually taught in several courses of a day or two each. Sessions on how goals are set, justifying capital investments, and handling the mechanics of capital requests are useful. Supervisory personnel are frequently taught advanced performance improvement skills, such as Six Sigma or the Toyota Production System. The human resources department often organizes these programs using faculty from planning, marketing, finance, and information services.

All associates are individually evaluated annually. Job performance reviews, "360-degree" (multi-rater) reviews, and learning opportunities help identify workers in three categories: promotable, capable, or improving. Workers who fall into the fourth class—incompetent—are usually warned, retrained, and either reclassified or dismissed. Improving workers are given extra training, mentoring, or counseling to move them to the capable category. Promotable associates are offered extra learning opportunities through special assignments, advanced training, expanded mentoring or coaching, committee responsibilities, and activities outside the organization. A career development plan, including learning goals and a program to achieve them, is jointly developed. Managers have explicit goals for developing their subordinates. These often include extra efforts to identify promotable members of underrepresented groups. Incentive compensation is awarded for fulfilling these goals in some organizations.

New entrants to management are evaluated closely. They have an initial period of enhanced training, sometimes called "residency" or "fellowship," that always includes mentoring and planned learning. The process is repeated as they mature, with increasingly challenging goals, building a reserve for higher management positions. (Some, of course, will leave for opportunities elsewhere.)

HRM designs the policies for identifying candidates and designs and administers the associate evaluation programs. Working with service units, it protects associate anonymity and ensures that all policies are administered uniformly and that there is always a clear route of appeal against actions the employee views as unfair. It trains managers in interpreting and presenting results and offers counseling.

Associate surveys combine elements of satisfaction and management evaluation. The surveys must be carefully worded and administered to ensure comparable and unbiased results. The 360-degree reviews allow evaluation by superiors, subordinates, and both internal and external customers. Associates leaving the HCO are interviewed. Their candid comments can be useful to correct negative factors in the work environment. HRM administers the interviews and presents findings to the appropriate managers.

WHAT IS SERVICE RECOVERY?

Service recovery is a program that empowers associates to compensate patients for service mistakes. Its primary purpose is to retain customer loyalty in situations where the organization has failed. Its secondary purpose is to create a record of unexpected events that can be used to identify and address opportunities for improvement (OFIs). When an associate feels that a customer has been treated in a substandard manner, she corrects the problem as fully as possible and is authorized to compensate the customer appropriately. Patients and families may be given flowers, free meals, free parking, even waiver of hospital charges, as indicated by the seriousness of the shortfall. All such transactions are reported in depth; these records identify process weaknesses and generate OFIs.

It is believed that service recovery improves customer satisfaction and reduces subsequent claims against the hospital. It has been proven cost effective in other industries. It is an extension of a long-standing procedure of "incident reports," specially handled written records of unexpected events. Because many of the events are clinical, it is a foundation for a more elaborate program of potential malpractice claims management, described in Chapter 5. The direct cost of the program can be managed with expenditure limits and required documentation. Its contribution is difficult to measure but almost certainly exceeds its cost. The program's success obviously depends on the organization's performance level. A hospital must have sound processes in place and a reasonable record of performance to make service recovery feasible.

WHAT IS THE ROLE OF INCENTIVE COMPENSATION?

An organization built on rewards and the search for continued improvement is strengthened by a system of compensation that supplements personal satisfaction, professional recognition, and team celebration with monetary bonuses. Excellent HCOs use a "gain-sharing" incentive system based on both strategic and unit performance and applied to the individual's work team. Gain-sharing requires annual negotiated goal-setting with primary worker groups. Goals are generally met, although major economic reversals may reduce or eliminate the bonus. The bonus may be wholly or partly tied to "stretch" goals that are more difficult to meet. Under gain-sharing, annual longevity increases disappear as incentive pay increases, and incentives provide a substantial portion of compensation, particularly for senior management.

Incentive compensation is subject to a number of documented difficulties. The key factors in recent successes are:

1. The incentive is based on achievement of both the operational (unit) and strategic (corporate) goals.
2. The measurement and benchmarking system for continuous improvement provides a rigorous foundation for negotiating goals and assessing progress.
3. The goals are almost always met and the bonuses earned. "Ninety-day plans" promptly address any part of the goals in danger of failure.
4. The goals are reset annually, keeping them consistent with strategic needs and technology.

WHAT ABOUT UNIONS?

The number of unionized hospital employees has been stable or declining for many years. The likelihood of unionization differs significantly by state, with the northeastern states and California most likely. Unions are likely to continue to be important in specific institutions and job classes but are unlikely to expand dramatically. Transformational management explicitly recognizes and responds to employee needs. It eliminates adversarial approaches and reduces the need for collective representation. It is successful in both union and non-union environments. Several excellent HCOs have extensive unionization. Managers must know the contract and abide by it, but whenever possible their actions should be governed by the goals of transformational management. Any distinction between unionized and non-unionized groups should be minimized. Management education helps them develop these skills.

CAN HRM DO CONTINUOUS IMPROVEMENT?

Much of HRM's improvement contribution is in collaboration with other units. Exhibit 11.2 shows typical OFIs and likely outcomes for HRM improvement. The department also prepares its own OFIs and goals and implements its own improvements. HRM measures its own performance using multidimensional measures (below). Most of both the collaborative and internal performance can be benchmarked against both healthcare and non-healthcare service organizations.

WHAT ARE THE HR AND HRM PERFORMANCE MEASURES?

HRM requires two measurement systems. Measures of the human resource, shown in Exhibit 11.3, are in every unit's operational goals. OFIs can be identified and pursued in specific units of the HCO or job classes. They are pursued collaboratively by HRM and the units involved.

An additional set of measures assesses the department itself, as shown in Exhibit 11.4. More than 250 metrics exist for various details of department operation, and consulting companies provide benchmarks and consultation services. Specific goals can be set and achieved by HRM.

The use of both metrics helps keep the contribution of the department in focus. Concerns are sometimes raised about the cost of human resources activity, which is substantially higher in high performing HCOs. The associate "learning" and "loyalty" that these costs produce must reduce the total cost of care.

Exhibit 11.2 Typical Improvements for Human Resources Management

Indicator	Opportunity	HRM Response
Potential RN shortage	Expand RN recruitment program	Install expanded part-time RN program, emphasizing retraining, child care, and flexible hours
High health insurance costs	Promote more cost-effective program	Revise health insurance benefits Install managed care Promote healthy lifestyles
Low incentive payments	Redesign incentive pay program	Expand eligibility for incentives, and improve measurement of contribution
Employee satisfaction variance	Identify common causes and address individually	Improve employee amenities Provide special training for supervisors with low employee satisfaction
Inadequate operational performance improvement	Support line review of causes	Form focus groups on motivation Seek evidence of worker dissatisfaction Review incentive programs
Labor costs over benchmark	Support orderly employment reduction	Curtail hiring in surplus categories Design and offer an early retirement program Start cross-training and retraining programs

HOW CAN AN HCO ACQUIRE HRM CAPABILITY?

Much of the "onstage" part of HRM must be at the HCO site, but many training elements are now Web-based. Much of the "backstage" support can be from remote central sources. This opens two

Exhibit 11.3 Measures of the Human Resource

Dimension	Measure
Workforce characteristics	Age, sex, ethnic origin, language skills, profession or job, training, certifications, etc.
Demand	New hires per year
	Unfilled positions
	Positions filled with short-term contract labor
Costs and efficiency	Labor costs per unit of output
	Overtime, differential, and incentive payments
	Benefits costs per associate, by benefit
	Human resources department costs per associate
Quality	Skill levels and cross-training
	Recruitment of chosen candidates
	Kirkpatrick scores
	Analysis of voluntary terminations
Satisfaction	Employee satisfaction
	Turnover and absenteeism
	Grievances

major sources of capability: centralized HRM in healthcare systems and HRM purchased from consultants. A health system central HRM can support planning, more elaborate educational programs, and a uniform information system with benchmarking. It can also promote consistent policies. Decentralized representatives available at each site concentrate on implementation. Similarly, human resources services can be contracted from outside vendors. The use of multidimensional performance measures makes contracting useful, and contracts can be arranged for specific functions or the entire human resources unit.

Exhibit 11.4 Measures of Human Resource Management

Dimension	Concept	Representative Measures
Demand	Requests for human resources department service	Requests for training and counseling services Requests for recruitment Number of employees*
Cost	Resources consumed in department operation	Department costs Physical resources used by department Benefits costs, by benefit
Human resources	The workforce in the department	Satisfaction, turnover, absenteeism, grievances within the department
Output/ efficiency	Cost per unit of service	New hires per year Hours of training provided per employee Cost per hire, employee, training hour, etc.
Quality	Quality of department services	Goals from measures of the workforce Time to fill open positions Results of training Audit of services Service error rates
Customer satisfaction	Services as viewed by employees and supervisors	Surveys of other units' satisfaction with human resources Employee satisfaction with benefits, training programs, etc.

*Employees receive many services from human resources automatically and thus are good indicators of overall demand for service.

SUGGESTED READINGS

Dell, D. J. 2004. *HR Outsourcing: Benefits, Challenges, and Trends.* New York: Conference Board.

Fried, B., and M. D. Fottler. 2008. *Human Resources in Healthcare: Managing for Success,* 3rd edition. Chicago: Health Administration Press.

Joint Commission, The. 2006. *Providing Culturally and Linguistically Competent Health Care.* Oakbrook Terrace, IL: The Joint Commission.

Studer, Q. 2004. *Hardwiring Excellence: Purpose, Worthwhile Work, and Making a Difference.* Baltimore, MD: Fire Starter Publishing.

Ulrich, D., and W. Brockbank. 2005. *The HR Value Proposition.* Boston: Harvard Business School Press.

Chapter 12 In a Few Words . . .

Every aspect of the environment of care must be designed and planned with the users in mind. The appearance of the facility often generates a patient's or an associate's first impression. Its convenience and functionality influence ultimate satisfaction. Signage should be abundant and unambiguous; grounds maintained and comforting; guest services friendly and helpful; and security present and effective. The HCO environment must also be prepared to handle natural disasters, large-scale accidents, and terrorist attacks.

Well-designed and well-maintained physical facilities and equipment improve efficiency, safety, guest comfort, and patient recovery. Smoothly operating food service, sanitation, maintenance, and materials management reduce waste and increase efficiency. Excellence in these areas supports improved financial performance through reduced cost per case and expanded market share.

Environment-of-care management often achieves these goals by contracting with specialized vendors. With either employed or contract associates, the keys to excellence are a transformational culture, measured and benchmarked performance, and continuous improvement.

Environment-of-Care Management

Is This Your HCO?

Your environment-of-care services get no serious criticism on surveys of patients and associates. Your supply chain has a few opportunities for improvement (OFIs), but it rarely fails or delays deliveries. The plant, the supply chain, and the disaster plan passed the most recent Joint Commission survey.

Nothing more to do, right?

Well, maybe. First check these questions:

How Do Excellent HCOs Surpass Ritz-Carlton?

Can you improve the patient response with more training for non-clinical service associates?
Have you nailed down all the ways an HCO is more complicated than Ritz-Carlton?

How Is Space Planned and Assigned? and How Does Design Improve Performance?

Have you optimized your space allocation?
Are you prepared to handle growth and replacement with 21st century design concepts?

How Does Environment of Care Tie to Risk Management?

> Are you capturing all "unexpected events," resolving them quickly, and learning from them to reduce future risks?

How Does the Environment of Care Improve?

> Are you near benchmark on all the measures listed in Exhibit 12.2?

How Do Environment-of-Care Services Control Cost?

> How much of your environment-of-care costs have moved away from allocated overhead toward actual transfer costs? See Exhibit 12.3.

What to Do Next?

HCO space needs change as technology and demand change. Not everything grows; some services shrink. How does the HCO take space away when it's necessary?
Your coach replies:

- Have a formal planning function. See "How Is Space Planned and Assigned?"
- Include the space plan in the board's annual review.
- Make sure there is an appeals process.
- Make sure there is a new use for the space that improves mission achievement.
- Try to soften the blow with equipment upgrades, refurbishing, etc.

Most environment of care is now provided by contractors who automatically become strategic partners. How does the HCO ensure a fruitful relationship?

Your coach replies:

- Uphold your contribution to the contract: space, equipment, training, and other services.
- Include performance measures (Exhibit 12.2), goal-setting, and continuous improvement as explicit clauses in the contract.
- Have a contract with annual renewal and extension, but explicit minimum standards.
- Periodically survey the market for alternate vendors, and share your findings with the contractor.

The point is not to cancel the contract, but to ensure that the contractor keeps up with best practice.

Environment-of-care management (ECM) operates essential facilities, supplies, equipment, security, sanitation, food service, and maintenance services. Its purposes are to:

- provide the complete physical environment required for the mission, including all buildings, equipment, and supplies;
- protect organization members and visitors against all hazards arising within the healthcare environment; and
- maintain reliable guest services at satisfactory levels of economy, attractiveness, and convenience.

The ultimate goals for environment-of-care services are easy to grasp:

1. The service rate should be 100 percent. The failure rate should be zero.

2. In as many encounters as possible, the "customer" (patient, guest, or associate) should perceive the services as "exceeded expectations."
3. The cost should be as low as possible after meeting goals 1 and 2.

Excellent HCOs in fact operate near 100 percent and frequently "exceed expectations." Their costs are not substantially higher than other organizations. They do it with careful planning, skillful performance measurement, contracting for many specialized services, and continuously improving operations.

HOW DO EXCELLENT HCOS SURPASS RITZ-CARLTON?

Ritz-Carlton, a 1992 Baldrige Award recipient and widely respected hotel chain, uses transformational and evidence-based management to provide excellent services. HCOs encounter a variety of problems that Ritz-Carlton does not. Here's a list of the major ones:

1. Like Ritz-Carlton, the HCO meets Occupational Safety and Health Administration and Environmental Protection Agency standards and their state equivalents. It also deals with hazardous materials and contaminated waste requiring specially designed systems, training for personnel, and drills for unusual threats.
2. In large HCOs, many more services operate 24/7. Electricity, methane, clinical gases, water, and sewage supplies are generally supported by redundant sources. Heating, ventilating, and air-conditioning services meet special air-handling requirements. Communications systems (Chapter 10) are also protected by redundancy.

3. Many more people move around in an HCO, increasing accident and crime risks. Employee education is helpful in promoting safe behavior and prompt reporting of questionable events. Security must be enhanced and coordinated with local police and fire service.

4. Many of the HCO's customers must be transported around the facility. The associates moving them should be trained in guest relations, emergency medical needs, and hospital geography.

5. An HCO's food service must be safe, appealing, and tasty, like Ritz-Carlton's. But it must also be inexpensive, and it should encourage good eating habits. Many HCOs also support home care and meals-on-wheels distribution.

6. In a natural or man-made disaster, Ritz-Carlton can help its customers and associates out of the building and shut it down. Many HCOs must have elaborate response programs, including training for associates and drills. The plans must include management of hazards; personal protective equipment; and clear assignment of tasks, locations, and training to prevent healthcare workers from exposure.

The "onstage" environment-of-care activities in excellent HCOs meet all these expanded requirements.

HOW IS SPACE PLANNED AND ASSIGNED?

Space allocation presents unique management problems. It has important symbolic, cultural, and marketing implications. Conflict over space is to be expected and must be systematically managed. Here's how excellent HCOs allocate space:

1. Forecasts of service needs are derived from the epidemiologic planning model and the needs described by service managers.

2. Service needs are translated to space needs described by location, special requirements, and size. Each unit seeking substantial additional space or renovation must prepare a request as part of a new program or capital proposal.

3. Space management is assigned to a single office. The office participates in new programs and capital budget review activities (see chapters 8 and 13), where most changes originate, and designs appropriate ad hoc review for other requests. The space management office prepares the facilities master plan, with assistance from operating units, internal consulting, and marketing staff.

4. Decisions allocating space are based solely on contribution to mission. The plan includes forecasts of specific commitments for existing and approved space; plans for acquisition of land, buildings, and equipment; plans for renovation and refurbishing existing space; plans for new construction; and anticipated costs.

5. There is provision for appeals to senior management, but appeals succeed only when the contribution to mission is clarified or expanded.

6. The facilities master plan is incorporated into the long-range financial plan and annual review and approval processes and is ultimately approved by the governing board.

7. The plant services department implements acquisition, construction, and renovation. Details of interior design are reviewed and approved by units that will be using the space. Financing is managed by the finance unit.

The strategy for preventing and resolving conflict makes sure that facts and the mission, rather than influence, determine the space allocation. It also ensures the financial success necessary to maintain the strength of the whole. There will still be winners and losers in space allocation, but the winners will document their contribution, and the losers will still have competitive, functional space.

HOW DOES DESIGN IMPROVE PERFORMANCE?

Better, safer, and evidence-based design environments prevent hospital errors, infections, and work-related stress. Private rooms, sound control, air quality, ecological impact, signage and information stations, wireless communication, and overall appearance are all important. A 2007 renovation of Bronson Methodist Hospital in Kalamazoo, Michigan, introduced many improvements, including art, light, and nature (such as a central garden courtyard), and helpful information technology (such as touch-screen kiosks).

Improved design is clearly an important component of a successful continuous improvement program. Spending on design innovations and upgrades can be recovered through operational savings and increased revenue.

HOW ARE CONSTRUCTION AND RENOVATION MANAGED?

Major construction and renovation usually call for extensive outside contracting. Recent innovations have emphasized turnkey approaches using a single contract. Advantages of speed and flexibility are cited, and it is likely that costs can be reduced if the HCO is well prepared and supervises the process carefully. Smaller renovation projects are often handled by internal staff with specific subcontractors.

Regardless of the size or complexity of the project, any project to change the use of space should be carefully planned in advance and closely managed as it evolves. A sound program includes the following:

1. Review of the space and equipment needs forecast
2. Identification of special needs
3. Trial of alternative layouts, designs, and equipment configurations
4. Development of a written plan and specifications
5. Review of code requirements and plans for compliance
6. Approval of plan and specifications by the operating unit
7. Development of a timetable identifying critical elements of the construction
8. Contracting or formal designation of work crew and accountability
9. Ongoing review of work against specifications and timetable
10. Final review, acceptance, and approval of occupancy

Involvement of end-users, especially caregiving associates and physicians, in planning and specifying the space requirements from idea conception to completion maximizes space functionality and stakeholder satisfaction and minimizes costly change orders.

HOW ARE ENVIRONMENT-OF-CARE SERVICES PROVIDED?

Specialized companies provide many environmental services under strategic partnerships or long-term contracts. Excellent HCOs incorporate partners into their culture and operations and maintain contracts that ensure continuous improvement. The services provided by employed associates can be viewed as contracts as well. In fact, they should be routinely compared to purchase from vendors and meet the same standards:

1. Contracts are designed to be ongoing but allow renegotiation at periodic intervals or in case of non-fulfillment.
2. Performance expectations are quantified in operational measures.
3. The contract identifies measures, methods of measurement, sources of benchmarks, and provisions for audit.
4. Contractors participate in annual goal negotiation and are expected to progress toward benchmark.
5. Procedures are established for empowerment and participation in process improvement teams (PITs), celebrations, and other events that make associates participants in the HCO's culture.
6. An HCO manager, reporting to or part of senior management, is accountable for maintaining the standards and responding to supplier needs.

These standards apply equally to internal and external suppliers. Under them, the current supplier is given a chance to improve, and usually does. Supplier change is not necessary because the supplier in place changes to do the job better.

The vendors and their associates cannot be viewed as outsiders. "Strategic partner" means "part of our team." PITs address many issues coordinating services between caregivers and environment of care. Each PIT must incorporate all of the involved services, regardless of contract status. PIT participation is valuable in three senses. First, the exchange of information leads to a better result, particularly with a skilled supplier that has experience at many HCOs. Second, suppliers gain insight into the underlying customer needs. They come away from the process understanding why the improvement was necessary and more committed to making it work. Third, participation is a reward. PIT assignments empower associates and provide an opportunity to reward effort.

HOW ARE HAZARDOUS MATERIALS MORE SAFELY HANDLED?

Clinical wastes, X-rays, anesthesia gases, some laboratory products, and some utilities and mechanical products present hazards to associates and guests. Following are four basic approaches to control of hazardous materials:

1. *Restricting exposure at the source.* Good design and good procedures for use reduce contamination risks. Special cleaning materials and procedures control hazardous material and speed recovery from spills and accidents.
2. *Training associates handling hazardous materials.* Associates are trained to safer behavior and encouraged to be vigilant.
3. *Attention to exposed patients, visitors, and associates.* An employee health officer examines any person believed to be injured or exposed to a hazardous substance. Appropriate treatment is provided without charge.
4. *Epidemiologic analysis of failures.* All failures and near misses are treated as unexpected events and reviewed in the HCO's risk management process.

WHAT IS THE "SUPPLY CHAIN"?

The supply chain concentrates most supply purchases under a materials management unit that implements the activities shown in Exhibit 12.1.

The best materials management achieves the lowest overall costs, rather than simply the cheapest price. Working with PITs and supplies users, materials management personnel strive to standardize

Exhibit 12.1 Materials Management Functions

Material Selection and Control	Processing
Specifications for cost-effective supplies	Elimination of processing by purchase or contract
Standardization of items	Improved processing methods
Reduction in the number of items	Reduced reprocessing or turnaround time
Purchasing	**Distribution**
Standardized purchasing procedures	Elimination or automation of ordering
Competitive bid	Improved delivery methods
Annual or periodic contracts	Reduced end-user inventories
Group purchasing contracts	Reduced wastage and unauthorized usage
Receipt, Storage, and Protection	**Revenue Enhancement and Cost Accounting**
Reduction of inventory size	Uniform records of supplies usage
Control of shipment size and frequency	Integration of clinical ordering and patient billing systems
Reduction of handling	
Reduction of damage or theft	
Economical warehousing	

items, reduce the number of different items purchased, establish quality criteria, and eliminate unnecessary use. They identify improved processes for supply use and new supply specifications. Clinical supplies are standardized through the protocol-setting process and the pharmacy and therapeutics committee. Materials management then negotiates prices, manages inventories, and maintains accounting records of use. Standardized materials, larger volumes, longer-term contracting, and competitive bidding allow better quality and reduce prices. Automation of inventories, ordering, and billing reduces handling costs and provides data for cost analysis. Most well-managed HCOs participate in group purchasing cooperatives that use the collective buying power of several organizations to leverage prices downward.

Most major vendors supply just-in-time service, effectively bearing the cost of inventory management. Vendors guarantee specific quality levels and are certified for compliance to International Standards Organization standards. Compliance eliminates the need for routine sampling of received goods. Centralized storage protects against theft and damage. Careful accounting and division of duties guard against theft and embezzlement. Some large vendors offer comprehensive materials management, providing a complete service at competitive costs. Some bulk supplies are delivered by robots to reduce costs.

HOW DOES ENVIRONMENT OF CARE TIE TO RISK MANAGEMENT?

Environmental safety is a part of the larger risk management program that develops a record of adverse or unexpected events from all sources: patient care, associate reports, security reports, events occurring to guests, events or potential events noted in rounds, and responsive listening. That record reflects evidence of the HCO's total exposure and measures the current level of safety. It is subject to reporting variation. As associates become comfortable with reporting and are convinced that the reports will be used to correct risks rather than punish reporters, the number of reports is likely to increase. The reports can be studied for commonalities such as locations, hours, or activities of unusual risk. The findings are OFIs.

A risk manager, sometimes called a safety officer, is charged with the responsibility to develop, implement, and monitor the risk program. A safety committee, which includes representatives of senior management, legal counsel, clinical services, and support services, can monitor the risk management process, protecting the culture and evaluating OFIs. OFIs are pursued in process-oriented PITs to preserve the blame-free culture. Corrections include process or protocol revision, equipment and facilities redesign, and expanded training for associates.

This approach has been repeatedly documented, most dramatically in commercial air traffic, where casualties have become extremely rare. It is highly cost effective, reducing malpractice litigation, associate lost time, and patient complications.

HOW DO HCOS PREPARE FOR EMERGENCIES AND DISASTERS?

"Disaster" is defined as any event suddenly increasing demand substantially beyond the HCO's normal capacity. When disaster strikes, even a large emergency service can face 20 times its normal peak load with little warning. The hospital may be inundated with visitors, families, and well-meaning volunteers in addition to the sick and injured. Normal channels of communication are often overwhelmed or inoperable.

The clinical response to mass casualties begins with triage, sorting patients according to needs for various levels of resources. The Centers for Disease Control and Prevention maintains a website of clinical information for both professionals and the public. It provides advice on treatment responses and mass casualty management (www.bt.cdc.gov/masscasualties/).

The elements of the response include:

- rapid assembly of clinical and other personnel;
- reassignment of tasks, space, and equipment;

- establishment of supplementary telephone and radio communication;
- triage of arriving injured;
- temporary shelter for homeless;
- continued care of patients already in the hospital;
- housing and food for hospital associates; and
- provision of information to press, television, volunteers, and families.

The American Hospital Association (AHA) maintains a disaster-preparedness website, www.aha.org/aha_app/issues/Emergency-Readiness/index.jsp. AHA identified additional areas that must be addressed to respond to terrorist activity:

- Communication and notification
- Disease surveillance, disease reporting, and laboratory identification
- Personal protective equipment
- Dedicated decontamination facilities
- Medical/surgical and pharmaceutical supplies
- Mental health resources

The need to convert spaces, enhance communication, expand supply distribution, and arrange utilities gives the facilities management department a central role.

Training for disaster is difficult, and results are uncertain. The plan must be tested as realistically as possible, and the test often uncovers substantial weaknesses. Once tested, the plan must be rehearsed periodically. Rehearsals should include drills with mock casualties and post-drill evaluations.

The hospital's response must be coordinated with other community resources. Police, fire, and public health organizations are immediately involved, and schools, churches, and businesses can be converted for emergency needs. A military-type command structure is necessary to reduce confusion and address rapidly changing situations. Government public safety personnel generally assume this role, under emergency powers. The Agency for Healthcare Research and Quality has tools for evaluating disaster drills, www.ahrq.gov/prep/drillelements/.

HOW DOES THE ENVIRONMENT OF CARE IMPROVE?

All environment-of-care services must first be reliable and safe, then satisfactory to associates and guests, and finally efficient. Satisfying customer requirements for quality and price must be the consuming objective. Examples of quality measures are shown in Exhibit 12.2. Joint Commission standards include a thorough review of structural measures of safety and emphasize environment-of-care planning, education, performance monitoring, corrective action, and evaluation. Inspections are critical to laundry, food service, supplies, maintenance, and housekeeping. Subjective judgment is usually required, but it is reliable when inspectors are trained and follow clear standards for cleanliness, temperature, taste, appearance, and so on. The frequency of inspection is adjusted to the level of performance, and performance is improved by training and methods rather than by negative feedback. Work reports—brief notes identifying specific events or issues—reveal correctable problem areas in plant maintenance and materials management.

Measures for the other dimensions of the operational scorecard are well developed and can usually be benchmarked from industrial sites or other HCOs. Demand is usually forecast by analysis of historical data on the incidence and duration of demand for each identified physical resource. Peak loads are frequently important. Human resources measures are similar to those in clinical and other support systems. Customer satisfaction measures recognize patients, guests, and internal customers.

Exhibit 12.2 Measures of Quality for Environment-of-Care Services

Type	Approaches	Examples
Outcomes	Technical standards	Many environmental services have explicit technical standards developed by organizations such as the National Institute of Science and Technology or the American Society for Quality.
	Unexpected event counts	Guest and associate accidents
		Delay and failure rates
		Service interruption rates
	Surveys	Guest and associate satisfaction
	User complaints	Service complaints
Process	Raw materials	Technical standards
		Compliance to purchase specification
		Failures and returns
	Service/product inspections	Food preparation
		Cleanliness
		Job completion
	Contract compliance	Return rates
		On-time supplies delivery
	Supply failures	Back-ordered items
	Inventory wastage	Losses of supplies
	Automated monitoring	Atmospheric control
		Power and utility failure
Structure	Facility	Life safety compliance
	Equipment	Elevator inspections
	Worker qualifications	Stationary engineer coverage

Benchmarks and scientific standards for these values are widely available. Numerous consultants offer information on labor standards for laundries, kitchens, and the like and cost standards for energy use, construction, renovation, and security. Competitive market prices are important benchmarks.

Environment-of-care work processes can be studied and improved by internal PITs, but most services are used by customers, who control the quantity of service used. A more elaborate system, which would include patient cooperation, is necessary to control costs.

HOW DO ENVIRONMENT-OF-CARE SERVICES CONTROL COST?

If environment-of-care services and products are "sold" to customers, control of the quantity of service is transferred to the end users. If the services are "allocated," the end users have no incentive to control quantities used. As shown in Exhibit 12.3, establishing a transfer price based on the unit cost allows an in-house "sale" that emulates a market purchase and substantially clarifies accountability. Transfer pricing has three important advantages:

1. The unit cost of producing the service can be benchmarked, improving the producing unit's goal-setting.
2. The unit cost can be compared to competing alternatives, such as purchasing instead of making the service, or centralizing producers for efficiency.
3. The consuming unit can benchmark the volume of service used and establish OFIs to optimize the quantity of service. (It is important to note that the "optimum" service is the one best fulfilling the user's mission, not necessarily the cheapest.)

Exhibit 12.3 Implications of Cost Accounting on Environmental Services

Costing Method	Impact on Producing Activity	Impact on Consuming Activity
Transfer pricing	Total cost per unit of service (TC/U) is calculated using activity-based costing. TC/U can be benchmarked. TC/U can be compared to competition.	"Buys" service and controls units consumed. Units per patient or customer can be benchmarked, established by protocol, or established by evaluating customer needs and satisfaction.
Allocation	Total direct cost (TDC) for producing activity is calculated. TDC can rarely be benchmarked.	Receives an allocated "indirect cost" charge for service. Indirect cost cannot be benchmarked. Consumer has no incentive to control use.

SUGGESTED READINGS

Joint Commission, The. 2009. *Environment of Care Essentials for Health Care,* 9th edition. Oakbrook Terrace, IL: The Joint Commission.

Joint Commission, The. 2009. *Planning, Design, and Construction of Health Care Facilities,* 2nd edition. Oakbrook Terrace, IL: The Joint Commission.

Ledlow, G. R., A. P. Corry, and M. A. Cwiek. 2007. *Optimize Your Healthcare Supply Chain Performance: A Strategic Approach.* Chicago: Health Administration Press.

Marberry, S. O. (ed.). 2006. *Improving Healthcare with Better Building Design.* Chicago: Health Administration Press.

Puckett, R. P. 2004. *Food Service Manual for Health Care Institutions,* 3rd edition. Chicago: American Society for Healthcare Food Service Administrators.

Chapter 13 In a Few Words . . .

Like knowledge management, many financial and accounting activities are "backstage," critical but technical contributions run by professionals. This chapter focuses on "onstage activities," the interaction of finance and accounting with other units of the HCO. These interactions occur in five major areas:

1. Annual environmental assessment and strategic goal-setting
2. "Roll-out" of strategic goals to individual operating units
3. Reporting performance versus goal
4. Analysis of process costs and proposed improvements
5. Preparation and competitive rank ordering of capital investment proposals

The long-range financial plan (LRFP) underpins many of these activities. It is a sophisticated, partially automated process that forecasts the HCO's financial future. Sound financial management, "backstage" except to senior managers and the governing board, makes the LRFP come true.

Accounting activities provide cost reports, cost analysis, and cost models to evaluate alternative future scenarios. Accounting's budget office manages the data for the goal-setting negotiations, coordinating a lengthy and complex process.

Audit activities protect all information—not simply financial information—from distortion and HCO assets against misuse and loss.

All of these activities are routinely measured and improved. The measures for "onstage" activities are a recent addition for most HCOs.

Financial Management

Is This Your HCO?

Cost reports come out on time. You reached agreement on the budget. The management letter from the auditor was clean. There's money in the bank. The LRFP suggests that the HCO can keep its A+ rating and meet its capital needs.

So, should your CFO get a raise? Not just for that. Challenge her with these issues:

Get better performance. See:

How Are the Strategic Goals "Rolled Out" to Operational Goals?
What's the Role of Cost Analysis and Forecasting?

Benchmark all the "overhead" costs, and get there. See:

How Can an HCO Control "Overhead" Costs?

Make sure capital expenditures deliver the planned return. See:

How Are Equipment and Program Opportunities Evaluated?

And, "Let's work together on the bond rating. The Performance Improvement Council (PIC) can improve our margin."

What to Do Next?

Your HCO is making good progress on its strategic score-card, but some opportunities for improvement (OFIs) are hard to translate to permanent improvement.

- Indirect costs are not moving to benchmark.
- The expected benefits are not achieved when the capital projects are completed.
- Some teams are struggling to reach their cost goals. Early reports suggest potential failure.

Your coach says financial management can help with all three of these:

Indirect cost management:

- Study best practices in other HCOs. Pay attention to services and customer satisfaction as well as costs.
- Move to transfer pricing (See "How Can an HCO Control 'Overhead' Costs?").
- Look for returns to scale. Consider merger or consolidation, or purchase from high-performing contractors.

Implementing capital expenditures:

- Focus on the capital request preparation.
- Make sure specific improvements in operating performance measures are clearly stated and accepted as a commitment by the operating team.
- When the installation's complete, the improved performance measures become goals.

Reaching cost goals:

- Act promptly to develop a "90-day plan" with the operating unit.
- The unit gets strong support from managers, internal consulting, and financial management.
- The plan could include re-setting the goal. More likely, it revises the process and retrains to correct the problem.

The purposes of the finance system are:

- **to record and report transactions that change the value of the firm;**
- **to assist operations in setting and achieving performance improvements;**
- **to provide financial analysis of new business opportunities, new programs, and large asset acquisitions to assist governance in strategic planning;**
- **to arrange funding to implement governance decisions; and**
- **to guard assets and resources against theft, waste, or loss and to guard the HCO's information against distortion.**

These purposes are accomplished through three organizational units—controllership, incorporating the first three; financial management, incorporating the third and fourth; and auditing, addressing the last.

Most of the functions supporting the purposes are "backstage." They are critical to HCO survival, and they are accomplished by finance and accounting professionals who also measure, benchmark, and improve their performance and report directly to senior management and the governing board. This chapter addresses the "onstage" contributions of finance, the places where it works directly with other units to improve their operations. Onstage activities center around:

1. The annual environmental assessment and strategic goal-setting
2. Negotiating annual operating goals
3. Reporting performance

4. Analysis of costs of current processes and proposed improvements

5. Preparation and competitive rank ordering of capital investment proposals

HOW DOES THE LRFP INFLUENCE THE STRATEGIC GOALS?

As noted in chapters 3 and 4, continuous improvement follows an annual cycle beginning with an extensive environmental review. The review (Chapter 14) is as comprehensive as possible and is led by senior management through its marketing and strategy team. It includes forecasts of the major operating parameters, such as discharges, surgeries, visits, and births. The assumptions are the critical element of financial planning. *Ceteris paribus* (other things being equal), extrapolations are not enough; critical variables must be thoroughly understood and carefully forecast. The forecasting process should include three specific protections:

1. Forecasts are obtained from respected and unbiased sources if available.

2. An effort is made to obtain alternate forecasts.

3. Sensitivity analysis is used to test the impact of alternative forecasts, and the implications of alternative forecasts are fully discussed.

These forecasts are incorporated into a long-range financial plan (LRFP), an automated model of expected revenues, costs, and sources of finance that can be used to model alternative strategies, identify capital needs, and justify borrowing. Once the governing board has identified its strategic direction, the LRFP also identifies profit requirements that must be translated to strategic cost and financial goals for the coming year. The board then establishes HCO-wide goals for the remainder of the strategic measures shown in exhibits 3.5 and 4.1—quality, patient and associate satisfaction, and efficiency.

HOW ARE THE STRATEGIC GOALS "ROLLED OUT" TO OPERATIONAL GOALS?

In large HCOs, several dozen work teams must "roll out" next year's strategic goals to each unit's operational goals, negotiating with the operating units to be sure the goals can realistically be achieved. The process is complex and repetitive. That's why it takes up to five months, as shown in Mercy's annual planning calendar, Exhibit 3.3.

As shown in Exhibit 13.1, goal-setting is separated from requests for capital and new programs. In goal-setting (the right hand side), each operating unit uses the strategic goals and its own continuous improvement to identify goals for all measures of its operational scorecards. The budget office supports the operating units with forecasts of unit activity; prices, trends, benchmarks, and competitor data; and overall corporate guidelines. The goal-setting process is managed by "packages"—specific bundles of information that are transferred from one unit or level to another. Timetables set deadlines for package transfers. The package concept allows the budget office to route coordinated information to multiple locations, permitting many different teams in the HCO to work at once. Automated models integrating multiple units support "what if" simulations, allowing the managers to explore a variety of alternatives. Units can experiment with alternative goal possibilities up to the package deadlines.

The best HCOs train managers how to approach the goal-setting and explore the implications of various answers three ways. First, hands-on training in using the software, support from superiors, and mentoring from experienced peers help first-line managers master their roles. Second, the board's budget guidelines are clearly explained. Each manager understands and

Exhibit 13.1 Integrating Strategic and Operational Goal-Setting

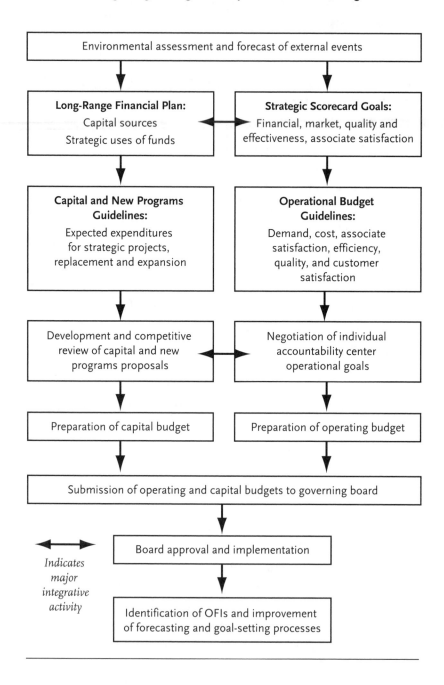

can explain to her team why the guidelines are important, how they were established, and how they were extrapolated from the organization as a whole to her unit. Third, the negotiations to reach the budget are considerate, fair, and realistic. This inevitably means that some units that are doing well will be challenged to excellence, while others that are struggling are given extra support.

These actions are a central part of transformational management. They are radically different from the top-down, authoritarian approaches of earlier management systems.

Several rounds are usually necessary. For the process to succeed, the following steps must be taken:

- The budget office must use the packages to coordinate critical forecasts across many units. For example, the expected demands for major service events and the expected prices for labor and supplies must be standardized across all units. The evolving needs must be identified as the rounds of negotiations proceed.

- The units must have effective, forward-looking improvement programs. The Performance Improvement Council (PIC) and the process improvement teams (PITs) established to meet last year's OFIs must have reached useful conclusions, ready to implement for the coming year.

- The PIC and all managers must review the results of each round and reach agreement on trade-offs between units.

- Goals must be truly negotiated, not imposed. Under transformational management, each team must understand its goals and have a clear plan to achieve them. Some organizations use two goals—one for minimally acceptable performance and a second "stretch" goal for exceptional achievement.

An excellent goal-setting process meets these measurable goals:

1. Line managers are convinced of the realism of the expectations.
2. Goals are almost always achieved.
3. Goals move closer to benchmark over time.
4. The budget process itself is subject to continuous improvement, becoming more rigorous over time.

HOW IS OPERATING UNIT PERFORMANCE REPORTED?

The budget office assembles goals and performance measures for each unit, for aggregates like service lines and clinical support services (CSS), and for senior management and the governing board. Actual performance data are assembled from several sources—accounting records, medical records, surveys, and unexpected event reports. The data reported exactly parallel the goals. Significance tests are shown on survey and clinical data. Color coding is used to flag values failing to reach goal. The best reporting systems have "drill down" capability. It is possible to go to source data—individual patient or employee records, or survey responses—to reconstruct each measure. Many measures can be accessed on demand through the intranet. Routine reports are generated biweekly or monthly. Some survey and quality measures are reported at quarterly intervals to increase sample size and reliability.

Reports are rarely a surprise to unit managers. "Red" and "yellow" values require formal 90-day plans to reach "green" by year end. These are developed by the unit managers and their superiors, often with assistance from internal consulting or other logistic services.

WHAT IS THE ROLE OF COST ANALYSIS AND FORECASTING?

Accounting personnel and internal consulting teams help PITs and operating units identify fruitful avenues of investigation, develop useful proposals, and translate operational changes to accounting and financial implications. PITs and units justifying capital or new programs often require detailed analyses and "what if" projections of resource implications. Common managerial accounting analyses include the following:

- Analyzing and forecasting interaction of demand, cost, output, and efficiency
- Comparing local production with outside purchase, often called "make-or-buy decisions"
- Comparing alternative protocols or work processes
- Ranking cost-saving opportunities to identify promising areas for efficiency improvement
- Preparing forecasts for expanding or closing units
- Developing goal expectations for new or expanded services when the operating conditions have changed

These applications are often complex technical exercises. Accounting and finance associates do the analysis. Success is usually a matter of clear reporting by the analysts, adequate discussion, and thoughtful response to questions. The operations managers' perspective can lead to important improvements in the modeling. Sensitive response to their questions increases their confidence in the results. Managers and senior managers see that all PIT members are comfortable with the assumptions and analyses and understand the implications of the findings.

HOW ARE EQUIPMENT AND PROGRAM OPPORTUNITIES EVALUATED?

Operational changes that require capital investment, such as new programs, facilities, or equipment, are separated from the operating budget, as shown by the left side of Exhibit 13.1. Isolating capital-related proposals facilitates:

- negotiation of operating goals, by simplifying comparison to previous years;
- more rigorous evaluation of proposed revisions;
- competitive review of capital opportunities; and
- specific implementation of goal changes related to accepted capital proposals.

The criterion for all capital investment is mission achievement. For the organization to thrive, new investments must always be selected on the basis of this criterion, which must balance various stakeholder needs. The process must identify the best proposals and seem predictable and equitable to associates. Here are the steps in the process:

1. As noted earlier, the governing board establishes a guideline for funds available for capital investment, based upon the long-range financial plan.
2. Ad hoc planning committees or PITs are commonly used to develop proposals. Early tests of benefit and cost are used to make sure a given proposal is worth the costs of proposal development. Only promising proposals are pursued.
3. Each of the service lines and major organizational aggregates rank proposals submitted within their activity. Managers ensure that all proposals get a fair hearing.
4. An executive-level committee with representation weighted to clinical systems integrates the rankings of the initial committees into a single list.

5. The planning and finance committees of the board review the rankings and recommend the list to be funded to the board.
6. As the approved projects are completed, the goals for the project are incorporated into the operating goals of the units affected. (Acceptance of a proposal automatically commits the unit to achieve the improvements used to justify the investment.)

The competitive evaluation is often led by internal consulting. Criteria for preparing and reviewing proposals are discussed in Chapter 14.

HOW CAN AN HCO CONTROL "OVERHEAD" COSTS?

"Overhead," the elements of cost routinely reported from general ledger transactions—including depreciation costs, charges for central services, and allocated central management costs—are always a source of contention. Operations managers deserve assurance that overhead is given the same level of scrutiny and rigorous control that their direct costs receive. Senior management should show that:

1. Costs of generating these services are accurately accounted and benchmarked.
2. Wherever practical, the best possible source of service is selected. This means outside vendors are used where appropriate.
3. Transfer prices and actual use of services, rather than arbitrary allocations, are used to develop the budget whenever feasible. Transfer prices give managers control over the quantities they use and can be compared easily to outside vendors.

4. Allocated costs are used only when necessary and are based on fair, reasonable, and consistent allocations.
5. Specific complaints are addressed promptly and thoroughly, and indicated changes are implemented.

IS AUDITING AN "ONSTAGE" FUNCTION?

Accounting, finance, and knowledge management are unusually susceptible to human failings—denial, avoidance, neglect, subversion, falsification, and theft. There is a constant risk that the HCO will let some matters slide, particularly when addressing them is likely to be unpleasant. The governing board and its audit committee are the first line of defense against this tendency. The internal and external audits, which are reported directly to the board, are essential elements of this defense. The board and senior management must provide full and visible support for the audits, including their independence and unique reporting relationship. Any threat to the integrity of the assets or the information must be promptly addressed. The culture must support thorough and judicious action on identified issues, avoid blame for honest error, and reward individuals who raise hard questions. This level of discipline promotes integrity. It reassures all associates and suppliers that their own actions will not be undercut by fraud, distortion, or carelessness. Contracts will be fulfilled; the data will be reliable; gaming will not be tolerated.

The discipline and the visibility make auditing an "onstage" activity. The auditors should be a visible presence. Their work should attract enough attention to reassure the committed associates and discourage those subject to temptation.

WHAT ABOUT REVENUE?

Under aggregate reimbursement contracts like diagnosis-related groups and ambulatory visit groups, few operating units have control of revenue. As a result, operating performance measures do not include either revenue or profit. Service lines that are large enough to have revenue and profit accountability should be monitored using the strategic performance measures, which include revenue, profit, and financial elements.

Revenue raises additional audit concerns. Much income is controlled by the diagnostic codes assigned. Assigning incorrect codes to increase severity ("upcoding") is illegal and should be monitored by both internal and external audit. Assigning too few codes or understating the severity of a condition is wrong as well, but the fact that the treating physician must attest to the codes under threat of criminal charge causes many physicians to understate severity. The solution goes beyond auditing to diagnostic coding assistance, including analysis of diagnostic and treatment orders to ensure capture of all treated diseases. The code selected is documented and justified. The solution also includes reassurance to the treating physicians. If the audit mechanisms and the criteria for adding diagnoses are understood and reliable, and specific queries are thoroughly discussed and evaluated, physicians will be confident and satisfied. Management's job is to see that both conditions are fully met.

CAN FINANCE/ACCOUNTING MANAGERS BE TRANSFORMATIONAL?

Under transformational, blame-free management, finance, accounting, and auditing associates must be seen as contributors and colleagues. They have too often been viewed as adversaries or enforcers. In large part, building constructive relationships is a matter of training and modeling. Finance personnel should be trained to fulfill Sharp HealthCare's 11 behavioral standards and five "Must Haves" (Chapter 2) as well as any other associate. The

CFO and the finance leadership must understand, implement, and model those behaviors.

The "onstage" interactions between finance and other managers are so widespread that they are almost constant. Those interchanges must be perceived by other managers as constructive. Clear, convenient systems and forms make routine information gathering as efficient as possible. Orientation and training sessions for finance personnel at all levels help them understand clinical procedures and participate in continuous improvement projects. Well-designed processes and training in consensus building make the interactions effective. It should be universally understood that operating management is responsible for setting, achieving, and departing from expectations. Finance personnel provide data and interpret them; they do not enforce budget discipline.

HOW IS ACCOUNTING'S "ONSTAGE" PERFORMANCE IMPROVED?

Finance and accounting, like every other unit of well-managed HCOs, must measure and improve its performance. Its "backstage" activities are extensively measured and benchmarked as described in finance and accounting texts. Exhibit 13.2 shows the array of operational measures that can be used for the "onstage" activity. These measures are entirely different from measuring the organization's financial position. They are much less commonly used, and unfortunately they are almost impossible to benchmark. Other HCOs rarely have comparable situations. Even without benchmarks, the Exhibit 13.2 measures can be used to identify OFIs, negotiate goals, and achieve continuous improvement.

Judging the right amount to invest in supporting other units can be challenging. For "onstage" interaction, effectiveness is more important than efficiency. Failing to meet user needs for reports and analyses can impair or endanger the HCO's overall program of continuous improvement. Excellent HCOs meet the following subjectively evaluated criteria:

- Reports and budget packages are clear, concise, timely, internally consistent, and consistent with external realities.
- Assumptions and their implications are specified.
- Prudent and reasonable sources are used to develop external trends, and a variety of opinions has been reviewed whenever possible.
- The report develops contingencies on major unpredictable future events.
- Unexpected events requiring modification are unforeseen by competitors and other external sources.
- The report is well received by knowledgeable board members and outsiders, such as consultants, bond rating agencies, and investment bankers.

Exhibit 13.2 Operational Measures of Accounting Services

Area and Examples	Goal	Benchmark
Demand		
Expected requests for services and hours required can be forecast from history	Timely and effective completion of transactions	Rarely available
Cost		
Costs of personnel can be identified and forecast from history	Fully meet customer needs without excess cost	Rarely available
Associate Satisfaction		
Satisfaction, absenteeism, and retention	Retention of all qualified associates	Provided by survey companies
Output/Productivity		
Requests completed and hours per request can be forecast from history	Timely and effective completion of transactions	Rarely available
Quality		
Can be assessed by outside consultant	Accurate reports, forecasts, and analyses Meet user requirements	Rarely available
Customer Satisfaction		
Surveys of user satisfaction	Develop "loyal" internal customers	User satisfaction can be benchmarked

SUGGESTED READINGS

Cleverley, W. O., and A. E. Cameron. 2007. *Essentials of Health Care Finance,* 6th edition Sudbury, MA: Jones and Bartlett Publishers.

Gapenski, L. C. 2009. *Fundamentals of Healthcare Finance.* Chicago: Health Administration Press.

Young, D. W. 2008. *Management Accounting in Health Care Organizations,* 2nd edition. San Francisco: Jossey-Bass.

Chapter 14 In a Few Words . . .

The internal consulting activity supplies essential knowledge for evidence-based management. It is a clearinghouse for any factual need arising in the HCO—particularly, needs emphasizing analysis. It completes an annual environmental assessment and maintains ongoing epidemiologic planning, benchmarking, forecasting, and statistical analysis. It responds to process improvement team (PIT) requests for information. It trains PIT members and HCO managers. It conducts specific analyses and models process alternatives for capital requests and strategic proposals. It facilitates legal, regulatory, and ethical reviews of changes. It coordinates all outside consultants. It manages change implementation and works to ensure capture of expected benefits.

Internal consulting must have senior management leadership, its own operational performance measures, and its own improvement function. Its customers—principally PITs—should be "delighted." It must maintain objectivity and empower the PITs and planning teams to make final decisions. It must earn its costs by the value of performance improvements. An increase in internal consulting expenditures must be justified by increased value of improvements.

Internal Consulting

Is This Your HCO?

Your Performance Improvement Council (PIC) has plenty of opportunities for improvement (OFIs), but a lot of them are just not discussed. "Too complicated," people say. "We can't do that here." Checking the ten functions of internal consulting (See "What's Involved in the Complete Fact Base for Decisions?"), an honest observer might say your internal consulting is failing its customers on most of them. But consultants are expensive and you certainly can't afford to hire full-time technical experts.

The solution is probably in the PIC, rather than in consulting itself. Try an HCO-wide stimulus campaign for OFIs. Identify the ones with the best near-term returns. Bring the units involved into the PIC meeting, and build quick-return road maps for each. The maps will show clearly how much is at stake and what specific resources are needed. They will justify spending some money or diverting some associates to new tasks, with an immediate return in view. Implementation of the projects starts a self-sustaining cash flow and allows the HCO to move toward the tougher OFIs.

What to Do Next?

Your HCO is on a roll. The number of OFIs is increasing. The PIC sorts them out. The best get implemented; the rest get sent back to improve or expand. The strategic scorecard shows handsome improvements. Most associates are "delighted" and they are taking home bonuses. But the senior manager for internal consulting says she's exhausted. "We're being run ragged. Not just me, my whole team."

Your coach says:

Don't ignore the problem! It will slowly stifle continuous improvement. You need a process improvement team (PIT) that includes senior management, logistics leaders, some clinical representatives, and possibly some board members to make sure you adequately support improvement activity. The motto is like the supply chain's —"the facts they need, when they need them, and sometimes before they ask."

The PIT could systematically review the ten functions and the 17 questions in this chapter. A better approach might be to look at the operational measures, Exhibit 14.4. Only a few can be benchmarked, but the PIT can evaluate the impact of improvement for most of them. An outside consultant, particularly one with a lot of experience in building internal strength, can help. (Note that the consultant usually has a conflict of interest—he sells what you lack.)

The purpose of the internal consulting operation is:

to provide information, forecasts, tools, and analyses in support of evidence-based management.

Under evidence-based management, operating decisions are analyzed by PITs and planning teams. Strategic decisions about the future of the enterprise are analyzed by the senior management team and the governing board. Internal consulting supplies the complete fact base for those decisions. The ideal is that even with complete hindsight, none of these decisions would be changed. Well-managed HCOs come closer to the ideal than others.

WHAT IS INVOLVED IN "THE COMPLETE FACT BASE FOR DECISIONS"?

The internal consulting operation is a clearinghouse for any factual need arising in the HCO, including analysis and forecasting of facts. The "any factual need" constraint makes the unit's accountability clear. It also reflects a critical limitation: internal consulting does not make decisions about proposals. It:

- completes an annual environmental assessment;
- maintains ongoing epidemiologic planning;
- provides benchmarking, forecasting, and statistical analysis;
- responds to PIT, senior management, and governance requests;
- trains PIT members and HCO managers;
- conducts specific analyses and models process alternatives for capital requests and strategic proposals;
- coordinates engagements of all outside management consultants;
- facilitates legal, regulatory, and ethical review of changes;
- manages change implementation; and
- works to ensure capture of expected benefits.

In addition, of course, it:

- measures, benchmarks, and improves its own performance.

HOW DOES INTERNAL CONSULTING WORK WITH CLIENTS?

Internal consulting has five major vehicles for helping its clients.

1. Immediate reply: a short answer, brief discussion, or short follow-up message.
2. Just-in-time support: training or a specific service, including coordinating support from other logistic and support services.
3. Designated team member: an internal consulting staff member assigned to the PIT.
4. Project team: a team of internal experts assembled from all parts of the HCO.
5. External consultants: consultants selected, instructed, and coordinated by internal consulting.

These vehicles have two important advantages:

1. Every client has a point of contact for technical support.
2. The client is the customer and has final say over the decision and the adequacy of the advice.

And two important consequences:

1. Any clinical or logistic support activity must respond to internal consulting's call for assistance.
2. Internal consulting controls outside consulting contracts.

The remainder of the chapter discusses specific contributions, internal consulting's "onstage" activities.

WHAT IS THE FACT BASE FOR THE ENVIRONMENTAL ASSESSMENT?

Internal consulting assembles an annual environmental assessment, including a detailed quantitative analysis, an analysis of qualitative information from boundary-spanning activities, and a written summary highlighting critical changes and opportunities. The report is widely circulated among the HCO leadership and provides background information for many PITs and planning activities.

Good environmental assessment takes into account the following:

- *Community demography, epidemiology, and economy.* All major trends in demographics and disease incidence, and forecasts to the future.
- *Patient and community attitudes.* Trends in healthcare purchases, sites, payment, satisfaction, and market share. Patient surveys, household surveys, complaints, and unexpected events. Results from listening, focus groups, direct interviews, and related sources. Benchmarks and major changes are noted.
- *Health insurance buyer intentions and health insurance trends.* Trends, prices, and market share of the various insurance products. The view of local groups on key matters such as services, debt, price, and amenities.
- *Trends in clinical practice.* Forecasts of major shifts in technology and the attitudes of practitioners and patients using the epidemiologic planning model if possible, otherwise qualitatively described.
- *Trends in associate supply and organization.* Important OFIs from the medical staff and workforce planning models.
- *Associate attitudes and capabilities.* Trends in the skills, attitudes, and compensation of current employees, physicians, and volunteers. Formal surveys are supplemented by focus groups and listening activities.
- *Progress on multi-year projects.* Status of ongoing initiatives and issues arising from the PIC activities.

- *Strategic OFIs.* Opportunities arising from the trend analysis and review of progress.

The annual review is a briefing book on the status of the HCO and its community. A summary highlights the most important issues, and the detailed review provides sources for further information.

WHO RUNS THE EPIDEMIOLOGIC PLANNING MODEL?

Internal consulting maintains the epidemiologic planning model (Chapter 3). The model itself is usually leased from a national consulting service. Internal consulting is responsible for local data inputs. It uses the model to produce short- and long-run forecasts for clinical demands and measures derived from them, such as employment, traffic, and supplies. The forecasts are used in human resources plans (Chapter 11), facility and service plans (Chapter 12), the long-range financial plan and the budget process (Chapter 13), the environmental assessment (this chapter), and strategic positioning (Chapter 15). Important forecasts should be offered with sensitivity analyses exploring alternative assumptions.

HOW DOES THE HCO FIND RELIABLE BENCHMARKS?

A high-performing HCO needs thousands of benchmarks. Internal consulting assists by collecting and evaluating benchmark alternatives. Benchmarking requires standard definitions of the measures being benchmarked and must be coordinated with information services. Benchmarking should include finding the best practice for a process. Benchmarks are frequently hierarchical, as "best in HCO," "best in system," "best in nation," and "world class." Hierarchy allows celebration of gains as they occur, while still making clear the opportunities for improvement.

HOW CAN USERS BE SURE PERFORMANCE MEASURES ARE RIGHT?

When operating team members and PIT members ask, "How do I know these numbers are correct?" a technical answer is called for. Standard definitions (Chapter 10) are the beginning. The statistical processes used to standardize are "backstage" and should be carried out or reviewed by a professionally trained statistician. They are as follows:

1. *Specification:* identifies subsets of the population or process, and calculates values for each subset. Day of week, shift, and season are common specifications for work processes. Gender, age, race, and education level often affect clinical demand. When these factors are outside the control of the operating team, variations they cause must be studied, and if possible removed.
2. *Adjustment:* uses specification subsets and calculates the value for a constant population, to allow "apples to apples" comparison.
3. *Forecasting:* incorporates the specification categories so that the total reflects their changes.
4. *Sensitivity analysis:* tests the extent to which a forecast will vary because of changes in the specification categories.

HOW CAN USERS BE SURE PERFORMANCE CHANGES ARE MEANINGFUL?

Statistical process control is a method of monitoring performance and identifying promising OFIs. Exhibit 14.1 shows a control chart with statistical control limits. The chart shows a statistically significant change in the underlying process at month 21, resulting in both a lower mean and less variation. It also shows that no subsequent month is statistically different from the current mean; the process is "in control." Study of a measure that is in control is not

Exhibit 14.1 Example of a Control Chart

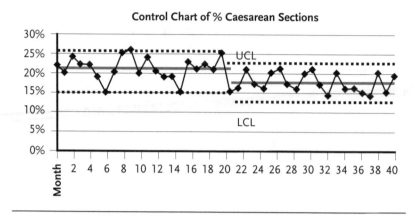

Control Chart of % Caesarean Sections

likely to reveal correctable process failures; a process in control is not a good OFI unless a benchmark can be found that is statistically significantly better than the current mean.

The applicability and design of statistical process control is also a "backstage" function, but one that can substantially improve identification and ranking of OFIs, leading to more effective results.

WHAT ABOUT LEGAL, REGULATORY, AND ETHICAL REVIEW?

Many performance improvement or planning projects raise complex questions of law and ethics, and some require regulatory approval. Internal consulting coordinates the services of the ethics committee, compliance office, and experts in environmental management and human resources management. It arranges appropriate regulatory approval.

Many larger HCOs also have an internal review board (IRB) that addresses questions related to the rights of patients in research situations. The IRB process is supervised by the Office for Human Research Protection (OHRP) of the U.S. Department of Health and Human Services. Concerns sometimes arise as to whether quality improvement activities are subject to IRB review. OHRP (www.hhs.gov/ohrp/qualityfaq.html#q2) has made clear that:

> . . . HHS regulations for the protection of human subjects do not apply to . . . quality improvement activities, and there is no requirement under these regulations for such activities to undergo review by an IRB, or for these activities to be conducted with provider or patient informed consent.

The OHRP definition of quality improvement activities is quite broad:

> . . . activities conducted by one or more institutions whose purposes are limited to: (a) implementing a practice to improve the quality of patient care, and (b) collecting patient or provider data regarding the implementation of the practice for clinical, practical, or administrative purposes.

HOW DOES INTERNAL CONSULTING IMPROVE LEADERSHIP?

Internal consulting provides basic training in continuous improvement to all members of the leadership group. New managers and promotable associates are offered short courses, usually one or two days each, in goal-setting, capital budgeting, and process analysis. These courses supplement training in supervision and meeting management (Chapter 11). They emphasize "how to" and actual examples, working simultaneously on analytic skills, interpersonal skills, and self-confidence.

Many HCOs offer advanced training in process improvement that emphasizes process control (Six Sigma), elimination of waste (Lean manufacturing), or integration of internal customers (Toyota Production System). The differences between these approaches may be more apparent than real; there is no evidence that any approach is superior. This training produces a cadre of trained managers so that most important PITs have several knowledgeable members.

HOW DOES INTERNAL CONSULTING HELP PITS AND STRATEGIC PROJECTS?

Internal consulting provides just-in-time training, an assigned adviser, or a consulting team as needed. Internal assistance brings a comprehensive knowledge of the organization that outsider consultants lack, and it is more directly invested in the results. As a clearinghouse for coordinating improvement efforts, it helps the PIC to coordinate multiple projects. Larger HCOs have substantial "backstage" skills, including activity-based cost analysis, regression analysis, econometric optimization models, simulation models, and other analytic approaches. Smaller HCOs can turn to consultants for these skills.

The improvement cycle calls for a pilot test of any proposed process revision. For simple changes, this may be simply a week or two of experience and a team meeting to review results, but for larger process redesigns, substantial field trials are appropriate. It is important to make the field trials as rigorous and objective as possible. Internal consulting is usually responsible for consulting on the experimental design, measures, and criteria. It is often used to analyze the data and make a recommendation, because it brings improved objectivity.

Strategic opportunities arise from the governing board and senior management. These often involve relationships with competitors and external stakeholders, and have consequences broader than the usual PIT. Examples include merger and acquisition opportunity, responses to competitor activity, and corporate restructuring. These proposals often present special needs for confidentiality and careful development of sensitive information. Although external consultants are often advisable, internal consulting can frequently help assemble necessary facts, develop forecasts, and identify implications.

HOW ARE CAPITAL INVESTMENT REQUESTS PREPARED?

Investments, such as new programs, facilities, or equipment, represent multi-year commitments to operational processes and programs as well as commitments of capital funds. Excellent HCOs have highly developed investment review systems to improve their investment decisions. The review process must select wisely, be prompt, be efficient, be perceived as reliable and equitable, and make sure that no reasonable opportunity goes unexamined.

Any investment concept or opportunity needs review against several conditions:

1. *Expected contribution to mission achievement.* This is usually measured by changes in operational goals, and for very large projects, changes in the strategic scorecard. The contribution, or return, must exceed the investment required.

2. *Physical constraints.* The project must fit space and utility constraints and meet safety requirements.

3. *Asset control and cost minimization.* Purchases must be carefully specified and, if possible, competitively bid.

4. *Implementation.* Installation must be scheduled and coordinated with ongoing activities.

5. *Actual contribution to mission achievement.* The expected contribution must be built in to the appropriate units' operational goals, and support provided to achieve the improved targets.

Most requests are programmatic, involving one or a few units. Well-managed organizations encourage programmatic proposals, because an abundant supply minimizes the danger that the best solution will be overlooked. Hundreds of programmatic concepts originate each year in large HCOs. Dozens survive initial review and are formally documented. Using a formal checklist of questions like Exhibit 14.2 increases objectivity and helps identify impractical projects quickly. Internal consulting ensures that the appropriate review has been completed.

Experienced managers soon learn the level of return necessary to gain funding. They drop or modify projects that fall short, reducing the set of proposals to a manageable group. Some projects are or become strategic and sufficiently complex to require direct board involvement, as described in Chapter 15. Strategic projects also benefit from the checklist in Exhibit 14.2.

HOW ARE CAPITAL INVESTMENT REQUESTS REVIEWED?

The review process shown in Exhibit 14.3 rank orders programmatic capital requests in broadening pools until there is a single list. The final list is presented to the governing board, which identifies how far down the list to fund based upon its annual goals. Board review of individual programmatic requests is rare and generally unwise. The board may examine the projects near the cut, moving up the list because proposals affected can safely be deferred to next year or down the list because the benefits of the next proposal are compelling.

Internal consulting manages the review process. (It can also be assigned to the budget office [Chapter 13].) The process emphasizes these elements:

- The operating unit is clearly responsible for identifying opportunities.
- The unit's senior managers act as advocates for the opportunities and coordinate support from other units, including internal consulting and clinical internal customers.
- Internal consulting assistance is readily available to develop proposals. It in turn calls on other logistic and strategic support. Information technology, human resources, environmental services, finance, and marketing are routinely involved.

Exhibit 14.2 Standard Questions for Evaluating Improvement Proposals

Mission, Vision, and Plan

- What is the relationship of this proposal to the mission and vision?
- Is this proposal essential to implement a strategic goal in the long-range plan?
- If the proposal arises outside the current strategic goals, can it be designed to enhance or improve the current plan?

Benefit

- In the most specific terms possible, what does this project contribute to healthcare? If possible, state the nature of the contribution, the probability of success, and the associated risk for each individual benefiting and the kinds and numbers of people benefiting.
- If the organization were unable to adopt the proposal, what would be the implication? Are there alternative sources of care? What costs are associated with using these sources?
- If the proposal contributes to some additional or secondary objectives, what are these contributions and what is their value?

Market and Demand

- What size and segment of the community will this proposal serve? What fraction of this group is likely to seek care at this organization?
- What is the trend in the size of this group and its tendency to seek care here? How will the proposal affect this trend?
- To what extent is the demand dependent upon insurance or financial incentives? What is the likely trend for these provisions?
- What are the consequences of this proposal for competing hospitals or healthcare organizations?
- What impact will the proposal have on the organization's general market share or on other specific services?
- What implications does the project have for the recruitment of physicians and other key healthcare personnel?
- What are the promotional requirements of the proposal?

Costs and Resources

- What are the marginal operating and capital costs of the proposal, including startup costs and possible revenue losses from other services?

Continued

Exhibit 14.2 *Continued*

Costs and Resources (Continued)

• Are there cost implications for other services or overhead activities?

• Are there special or critical resource requirements?

• Are there identifiable opportunity costs associated with the proposal, or other proposals or opportunities that are facilitated by this proposal?

• Are there other intangible elements (positive or negative) associated with this proposal?

Finance

• What are the capital requirements, project life, and finance costs associated with the proposal?

• What are the competitive price and anticipated net revenue?

• What are the demand elasticity and profit sensitivity?

• What are the insurance or finance sources of revenue, and what implications do these sources raise?

• What is the net cash flow associated with the proposal over its life, and the discounted value of that flow?

Other Factors

• What are the opportunities to enhance this proposal or others by combination?

• Are there customers or stakeholders with an unusual commitment for or against the proposal?

• Are there any specific risks or benefits associated with the proposal not elsewhere identified?

• Does the proposal suggest a strategic opportunity, such as a joint venture or the purchase or sale of a major service?

Timing, Implementation, and Evaluation

• What are the critical path components of the installation process, and how long will they take?

• What are the problems or advantages associated with deferring or speeding the implementation?

• What are the anticipated changes in the operating budget of the units accountable for the proposal? What changes are required in supporting units?

Exhibit 14.3 Programmatic Capital Review Process

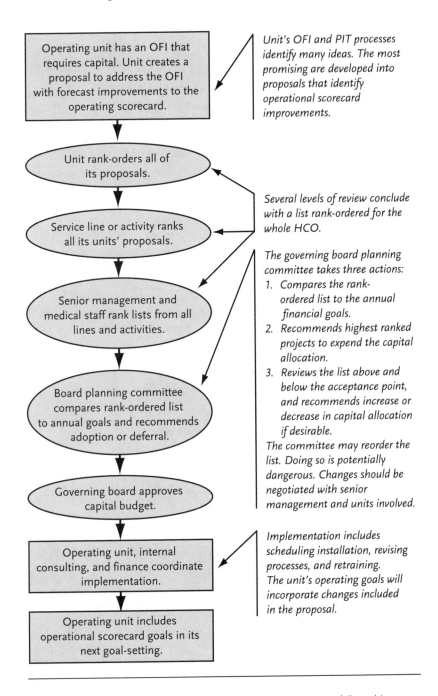

Operating unit has an OFI that requires capital. Unit creates a proposal to address the OFI with forecast improvements to the operating scorecard.

Unit's OFI and PIT processes identify many ideas. The most promising are developed into proposals that identify operational scorecard improvements.

Unit rank-orders all of its proposals.

Service line or activity ranks all its units' proposals.

Several levels of review conclude with a list rank-ordered for the whole HCO.

Senior management and medical staff rank lists from all lines and activities.

The governing board planning committee takes three actions:
1. *Compares the rank-ordered list to the annual financial goals.*
2. *Recommends highest ranked projects to expend the capital allocation.*
3. *Reviews the list above and below the acceptance point, and recommends increase or decrease in capital allocation if desirable.*

Board planning committee compares rank-ordered list to annual goals and recommends adoption or deferral.

The committee may reorder the list. Doing so is potentially dangerous. Changes should be negotiated with senior management and units involved.

Governing board approves capital budget.

Operating unit, internal consulting, and finance coordinate implementation.

Implementation includes scheduling installation, revising processes, and retraining. The unit's operating goals will incorporate changes included in the proposal.

Operating unit includes operational scorecard goals in its next goal-setting.

- Costs and benefits are quantitatively documented in the proposal, and the unit agrees to the benefits as future operational scorecard goals.
- The HCO's mission statement and its commitment to evidence-based medicine and evidence-based management are used as the guide to rank new opportunities.
- There is medical and nursing review and ranking of all projects with clinical implications.
- Clinical and non-clinical proposals are judged competitively with one another, in a common review process that includes medical and clinical support service representation.

Consistency is the hallmark of success. In most HCOs, there is always somebody claiming an urgent need to make exceptions to the review process. Organizations that yield often to these pleas soon discover that the exceptions undermine the process. At that point, political influence and persuasive rhetoric become the criteria that guide investments.

It is important to note that the planning staff never judges the proposals themselves. They provide facts and concepts to managers and let them decide. They protect the process of review itself, discouraging attempts to subvert or avoid it and making the preparation as efficient and fair as possible.

HOW ARE NEW PROGRAMS IMPLEMENTED AND INTEGRATED?

Once new processes or capital investments are recommended for adoption, two further steps are required:

1. Implementation: Project management can substantially reduce both costs and delays. The use of PERT (program evaluation and review technique) software to coordinate multiple contributions can save millions in large projects.

2. Integration: Each proposal is accepted because it promises specific performance improvements. Those promises must be built into the operating goals of the units involved. Progress toward them must be monitored, and assistance arranged if difficulties are encountered.

The implementation of projects requiring construction or extensive renovation is commonly assigned to environment-of-care management (Chapter 12). Smaller projects are often monitored by internal consulting. In both cases, internal consulting monitors the goal-setting process to ensure that the claimed benefits are achieved.

WHY SHOULD INTERNAL CONSULTING MANAGE ALL OUTSIDE CONSULTANTS?

Many HCOs use commercial consultants, consortiums such as VHA, and consultation from the central offices of larger systems. Outside consultants have the advantage of drawing on similar problems elsewhere and often have developed specialized tools and solutions that have a demonstrated record of success. Assigning contracting authority to internal consulting encourages coordination, sustains the clearinghouse knowledge, and maximizes the benefit from the consulting engagement. The keys to successful use of external consultants are the following:

1. The assignment should be clearly specified in terms of process, timing, and goal. It is sometimes wise to use consultants for general education and to gain fresh insights into vague, ill-defined problems, but such use should be limited to short-term assignments.
2. Internal skills and knowledge should be fully utilized before external consultants are engaged, and internal experts should work directly with external experts. This minimizes cost and maximizes retention of the external advice.

3. Consultant firms should be selected on the basis of relevant prior experience. In the absence of direct experience with a consultant, opinions of other clients should be solicited before any major engagement.

4. Consultant activities should be carefully monitored against the specifications throughout the project. A timetable and monthly interim achievement checkpoints should be used.

5. Each consultant must have an explicitly assigned internal supervisor. Failure to identify a point of contact slows the consultants, adds to their costs, and defeats the possibility of continuous monitoring during the contract period.

HOW DO THE PITS KEEP CONTROL OF THE DECISIONS?

"We'll study that," is a common response in all kinds of negotiations. It is often the correct response, but empowerment requires that the study be conducted fairly and expeditiously. Using the study as a way to avoid the decision or forward a special interest is destructive. This imposes three duties on the PIC and internal consulting:

1. Scrupulously maintain their commitment to the evidence, making sure that it neither conceals nor distorts any alternative fact, analysis, or proposal.

2. Ensure appropriate representation on each PIT or planning committee—no unit with a stake in the outcome can be omitted—and a level playing field among members.

3. Enforce the timetable so that the PIT proceeds in a timely manner.

These are matters addressed by the charge, membership, and timetable that the PIC establishes for each PIT.

Sophisticated measurement and analysis make it easy for internal consulting to exercise excessive or improper influence over the final decisions. Any PIT or operating team member has the right to understand:

- *What:* definition, provenance, and limitations of all the measures that are used in an analysis.
- *Why:* the implications of alternative measures.
- *How:* the limitations of the analytic process and the implications of alternative processes.

The consultant team must address these issues directly. A question on the client survey, "How often did internal consulting *explain things* in a way you could understand?" will monitor performance. (The wording and the emphasis are taken directly from the HCAHPS patient survey.)

HOW MUCH SHOULD INTERNAL CONSULTING COST?

It is notable that there is no benchmark for operating cost of internal consulting. As is true of all logistic services, the optimum cost is not what some other HCO pays, but the expenditure that yields maximum return on strategic performance. Internal consulting must cover its cost with operating improvements. An HCO bears an indirect cost burden for the internal consulting service. To succeed, it must increase net income using some combination of increased revenue and decreased costs.

As of 2009, the trend was increasingly clear. The high-performing HCO makes a substantial investment in its informtion, human resources, environmental services, financial, internal consulting, and marketing capabilities. It uses the total investment to attract patients and caregivers and increase market share. The underlying business model is as follows:

- Operate in a patient-friendly manner, with better hours, responsive caregivers, prompt service, attractive amenities, and high quality of care.
- Operate in a caregiver-friendly manner, with empowerment, rewarding values, reliable logistics, and performance incentives.
- Operate efficiently, using improved processes to eliminate waste and higher volumes to reduce unit costs.
- Operate effectively, avoiding unnecessary treatment and promoting overall health, so that insurers are willing to pay more for each unit of treatment.
- Move toward benchmarks on the strategic scorecard.

Failure to meet any of these conditions is an OFI, subject to investigation and improvement by the PIC and the internal consulting unit.

HOW CAN INTERNAL CONSULTING BE IMPROVED?

Under the ongoing guidance of internal consulting, the HCO as a whole develops an ability to identify, understand, and react to opportunity. That ability becomes a major competitive advantage and a strong bulwark for evidence-based management.

Internal consulting maintains an operational scorecard (see Exhibit 14.4). It makes a systematic effort to benchmark itself wherever possible and to identify and achieve best practices. It is fruitful to view internal consulting as an independent subsidiary, operating as though it were an outside consulting company. That approach leads to an "engagement" mentality on the part of the

Exhibit 14.4 Operational Performance Measures for Internal Consulting

Dimension	Measure	Example
Demand for services	Counts of user requests Projects initiated or assigned Unfilled or delayed requests	Log of requests and assignments Delays to respond to service requests
Cost	Total direct costs Hours on assigned projects External consultant costs Data and information acquisition costs	Personnel hours assigned to projects External consultant fees Costs of comparative or benchmark information
Human resources	Satisfaction scores of internal consulting personnel Vacancy rates and turnover	Surveys, personal and group discussions of work environment
Productivity	Total cost as percent of HCO operating cost Cost per support request Cost per project completed Total cost as percent of improvements implemented	"Contribution," actual improvements in operational measures from completed projects compared to annual internal consulting costs
Outcomes quality	Forecast accuracy: variation from actual Timeliness: projects completed on schedule Improvements achieved	Variation of annual forecasts from actual Accuracy of epidemiologic planning model forecasts Counts of projects completed on time Counts of projects achieving expected goals
Client satisfaction	User satisfaction surveys Overall planning service Project-specific service: Recognition and resolution of problems Supportive attitude	Users' responses to services: "would rehire, would recommend"

team members. They must keep logs of activities, and individual effort must be transfer priced to show direct costs per project. Once this is done, it is possible to track consulting costs, proposal decisions, projected improvements, realized improvements, and client satisfaction. Although some measurements will be estimates, even approximations will be useful.

The outcomes quality and customer satisfaction measures on the operational scorecard are important indicators of the success of these values; any deterioration is an immediate OFI. Careless or incomplete work by internal consulting can fatally disable an HCO. Successful planning units excel in four areas. They:

1. take extra pains to guard against oversights,
2. use the best comparative data and the most objective forecasts they can obtain,
3. are rigorous in their evaluation of costs and benefits, and
4. work consistently to "delight" their internal customers.

An outside review team can be helpful in identifying specific areas that need improvement. Internal reviews, where a work product by one analyst is critiqued by a second, are also important and should be routine on all large-scale projects. Attendance at technical training programs allows analysts to keep and expand their skills. The visible commitment of the senior management leader is important. Individual performance reviews are also useful and can be tied to incentive compensation.

SUGGESTED READINGS

Alemi, F., and D. H. Gustafson. 2009. *Decision Analysis for Healthcare Managers.* Chicago: Health Administration Press.

Ozcan, Y. A. 2009. *Quantitative Methods in Health Care Management,* 2nd edition. San Francisco: Jossey-Bass/Wiley.

Porter, M. E. 2008. *On Competition.* Boston: Harvard Business School Publishing.

Sproull, R. 2009. *The Ultimate Improvement Cycle: Maximizing Profits Through the Integration of Lean, Six Sigma, and the Theory of Constraints.* New York: Productivity Press.

Chapter 15 In a Few Words . . .

Marketing and strategy are intertwined activities relating the organization to all its stakeholders, including competitors. Marketing includes identification and segmentation of exchange partners, extensive listening, branding, promotion to customers and associates, and management of relations with competitors and other community agencies. In strategy, the governing board selects the organization's direction and relationships, positioning the organization through its mission, values, services, and partnerships. Extensive stakeholder discussions identify, prioritize, and implement strategic opportunities. The managerial role emphasizes the leadership necessary to keep large groups of people with inherently conflicting agendas aligned toward the mission. Alignment is achieved through the tools for continuous improvement, the processes for building consensus, and continuing rewards. Success builds on itself.

Marketing and Strategy

Is This Your HCO?

With 1,300 employees and a budget of $70 million, you are close to the median U.S. general hospital. Logistic services—IT, HR, plant, finance, and internal consulting—consume over $20 million a year, and there's plenty of griping about it. The associates in those units are loyal, dedicated, and overworked. The opportunities for improvement list for these units is a mile long, and getting longer, because the units put all their energy into helping the caregivers and clinical support teams.

The solution won't be easy, but here's the core of it:

1. Check your clinical outcomes: cost per case, length of stay, complications, unexpected events, and market share. These are the main drivers that pay for more logistic services. If they aren't benchmark for organizations your size, find the most promising logistics OFIs and develop and implement a solution plan.
2. When your clinical operations push benchmark, the next step is a larger scale operation. There are three basic approaches:
   a. Find reliable consulting companies that offer a competitive retainer price and can provide you with the skills you need for your logistic OFIs.

b. Merge with a system that can document excellence on the strategic scorecard (Exhibit 3.5); show your board how it can move your HCO to the next level; and expand your logistics resources.

c. Acquire another HCO and use your team as core for an expanded operation.

By focusing your annual retreat and board education program on the shortfall from benchmark and the OFI list, you can help the board and clinical leadership understand the issues and the solution.

What to Do Next?

Your coach says you can put any HCO in one of the following categories. The strategic path for each should consider some specific issues.

1. *Your HCO is a sole community hospital.*
   Think about enhancing your clinical and logistic capability through a merger or partnership with a high-performing larger system. These days, with telemedicine and electronic communication, a "big brother" isn't all bad.
   Think about community health (Chapter 9). You and your associates are the de facto health leaders. Move your community to benchmark on the community health measures (Exhibit 9.5).

2. *Your HCO competes with others, and its market share is stable.*
   Think about Jack Welch's advice, "If you're not number one or number two, fix it; sell it; or close it." Which solution fits depends upon clinical performance. If your clinical measures are near benchmark, there's a fourth option: acquire the weakest competitor.

3. *Your HCO competes with others, and its market share is declining.*
   Welch would fix it. If he couldn't fix it, he'd merge it, or find a strong partner. If he couldn't fix it or merge it, he'd close it.

The HCO described in the preceding chapters thrives only because it fulfills the changing needs of stakeholders, as the stakeholders perceive them. The purpose of marketing and strategy is

to identify, evaluate, and respond to changes in stakeholder needs.

Marketing is the deliberate effort to establish fruitful relationships with exchange partners and stakeholders. Strategy is the selection of the scope of services, the profile of stakeholder needs to be met. In successful HCOs, marketing and strategy are a seamless, continuous activity that monitors and modifies the basic direction of the enterprise and, in some cases, redirects the enterprise through merger, acquisition, or closure.

WHAT ARE THE TECHNICAL REQUIREMENTS OF MARKETING AND STRATEGY?

A successful HCO strategy must meet several different and interrelated criteria:

1. The services offered use processes that are competitive on cost, amenities, and quality.
2. Demand for services is adequate to cover the fixed costs and meet quality standards.

3. The work environment attracts and retains associates who are committed to implementing the strategy.
4. The services identify and capitalize on a competitive advantage, a reason customers select the HCO over alternatives.
5. The constellation of services attracts and builds patient and associate loyalty and fulfills the realistic expectations of patients and associates.

Each of these criteria presents a risk of failure. Only the first criterion is attacked solely by improving the processes within the organization itself. All the rest require attention to the whole. The technical functions that support them are described in Exhibit 15.1.

WHAT IS MARKETING? IS IT JUST PROMOTION?

The term "marketing" has a professional definition that is substantially broader than the common use of the term:

the analysis, planning, implementation, and control of carefully formulated programs designed to bring about voluntary exchanges of values with target markets for the purpose of achieving organizational objectives.[1]

Others use a "four Ps" mnemonic to capture the breadth of the concept:

Product: What exactly is the product or service offered in the exchange? (includes benchmarks and competitive operational standards)
Place: Where and how does the exchange take place? (includes hours of service, geographic locations, and relations between services)

---

[1]Kotler, P., and R. N. Clarke. 1987. *Marketing for Health Care Organizations,* 5. Englewood Cliffs, NJ: Prentice-Hall.

Exhibit 15.1 Functions of Marketing and Strategy

Function	Processes	Purpose
Marketing		
Identify and segment customer and associate markets	Surveillance, data analysis, segmentation of market	Understand stakeholder needs and identify participants whose needs are consistent with the HCO mission.
Listen to exchange partners' needs	Surveys, focus groups, monitors, personal contact	Gain a clear and complete understanding of what the HCO must do to attract exchange partners in sufficient number.
Develop brand and media relations	Communication to establish awareness of HCO and its scope of services	Make the HCO as a whole attractive to the community by emphasizing widely shared goals through a variety of communication methods.
Persuade potential customers to select the HCO's services	Communication to patient populations with specific needs	Make potential patients aware of the services and persuade them to select the organization over its competitors.
Attract and motivate capable associates	Communication to target associate populations, advertising, incentives	Ensure a steady stream of qualified applicants, even in areas of personnel shortages.

Continued

Exhibit 15.1 Continued

Function	Processes	Purpose
Marketing (Continued)		
Manage other stakeholder relationships	Surveillance, senior management listening, partnerships to align other stakeholders	Establish constructive relationships with other organizations, such as insurance intermediaries, employers, and providers of competing or complementary services.
Improve the organization's marketing activity	Marketing plans, goal-setting, evaluating marketing effectiveness	Set goals that move toward benchmarks and values for market share.
Strategy		
Maintain the mission, vision, and values	Visioning exercises	Allow multiple stakeholders to consider and comment on mission, vision, and values.
Define the strategic position	Evaluating and selecting alternative approaches to maximizing mission achievement	Position an array of clinical services geographically to achieve a competitive advantage with an identified population.
Document the strategic position	Maintaining and coordinating strategic plans	Integrate multiple strategic and programmatic responses.
Implement the strategic position	Managing investments and processes that will achieve the strategic goals	Ensure that the HCO responds to opportunities and threats arising from external events.
Improve strategic process	Establishing goals and OFIs for strategy processes	Continuously improve strategy and strategy formulation.

Price: What is the total economic value of the exchange? (not only the price paid the vendor but also collateral costs such as transportation and lost income)

Promotion: What activities are necessary to bring the opportunity to the attention of the stakeholders likely to accept it? (includes publicity, advertising, incentives)

The order of the four Ps is important. The consequences of bad product design or placement cannot generally be overcome by low prices or extensive promotion.

WHY SEGMENT MARKETS?

Market segmentation differentiates exchange partners into particular subgroups based on the group's exchange need and the message to which they will respond. It is similar to statistical specification (Chapter 14). Along with listening and branding, it underpins the other marketing functions. People of different ages and genders have different healthcare needs, use different insurance, want different schedules and amenities, and listen to different media. Efforts that are not segmented are inherently inefficient.

HOW DOES AN HCO LISTEN TO STAKEHOLDERS?

Excellent HCOs use all the major listening approaches summarized in Exhibit 15.2. Many reports yield qualitative rather than quantitative information. The marketing unit plays a critical role in assembling and interpreting these data.

Leading HCOs now expect managers to report learning from all kinds of contacts, including rounds, on-call issues, and contacts with outside groups and organizations. "Incident" or "unexpected event" reports, service recovery reports, and various complaint vehicles generate qualitative information, as do "exceptional effort" or "caught in the act" cards. The reports are a major information source for risk management, but they also reveal marketing opportunities. Underreporting is a serious issue. Associates are trained to report service-recovery situations and clinical errors whenever they occur. Managers are trained to avoid blame. Follow-up rewards reporting and focuses on prevention. Statistical monitors can be constructed around event counts. Their most important use is to validate the subjective reporting processes.

WHAT IS BRANDING?

Branding maintains the overall reputation or image of the organization and conveys its competitive advantages. Branding activities include public and community relations, image advertising and promotion, maintenance of an attractive website, and media relations. A branding program includes descriptive information for various media; relationships with other influential community agencies, such as schools and the faith community; and sponsorship of community events, such as health fairs and athletic teams. It also includes personal appearances by management and caregivers, deliberate contacts with community influentials and opinion leaders, and damage control for negative media events. An increasing number of HCOs release specific information about finances, service, and quality, documenting their achievements.

Branding is far from a panacea. It takes a large number of exposures simply to increase name recognition, and changing attractiveness is harder. At the same time, an established reputation—being among the first two or three names people independently recall for healthcare—is a valuable asset, hard to replace, and well worth protecting.

Exhibit 15.2 Major Listening Activities

Activity	Description	Application
Formal Surveys		
Patient satisfaction	Telephone, Web, or mail survey	Offered to inpatients and various categories of outpatients
		Assesses satisfaction with amenities and perceived quality of care
		Forms the basis for the "loyal" patient estimates
		Usually provided by a national survey firm, which supplies comparative data and evaluates reliability
Associate satisfaction	Telephone, Web, or mail survey	Offered to various categories of associates
		Forms the basis for the "loyal" associate estimate
		Usually provided by a national survey firm, which supplies comparative data and evaluates reliability
Community	Telephone or mail survey	Estimates market share, prevalence of insurance, travel patterns, and other characteristics not in the decennial census
		Can be used to update census data
		Can be focused on specific population segments

Continued

Exhibit 15.2 *Continued*

Activity	Description	Application
Monitors		
Unexpected event reports	Associate-generated written reports	Associates are encouraged to report any event that represents a serious failure, such as a fall, a clinical error, or an unacceptable delay; gifts to patients under service recovery programs require reports.
Service recovery	Written reports of actions to correct failures	Associates are authorized to offer gifts or benefits in cases where processes have egregiously failed; the incident and the recovery must be reported in writing.
Complaints	Written, oral, or electronic reports from patients or associates	Patients are offered "bounce-back" cards, and both patients and associates are encouraged to communicate directly with organizational authorities.
"Caught in the act"	Written reports of exceptional behavior by associates	Cards for "caught in the act" are publicly available; the events reported are judged by a panel, and prizes are awarded.
Statistical process control	Counts of untoward events documented in the patient record	The electronic record can be surveyed for evidence such as diagnoses, specific drug orders, progress notes, or treatments reflecting adverse events such as infections, falls, treatment errors, and complications. These can be tracked and monitored either as sentinel events (all cases investigated) or using statistical process control (Chapter 14).

Exhibit 15.2 Continued

Activity	Description	Application
Personal Contact		
Focus groups	Small groups of current or potential customers meeting face-to-face	Focus groups are encouraged to speak candidly about existing services and explore what is important about proposed services; they provide insight to specific process opportunities that do not arise in surveys.
"On-call" managers	24/7 designated contact official	A senior manager is always accessible to patients or associates for prompt attention to complaints or difficulties; this allows direct intervention and service recovery in complex situations.
Walking rounds	Regularly scheduled senior management visits	Personal contact and visits to actual work sites by front-office managers; these visits encourage questions, explain positions, reward efforts, validate public pronouncements, and humanize.
Shadowing and walk-throughs	Observation of a single patient through a complex process	Shadowing allows associates to understand the process and its impact on patients; walk-throughs actually duplicate patient activity.
Mystery shopping	Observation of a competitor's process	Mystery shoppers were initially used to discover competitors' prices. In healthcare, they reveal competitors' processes and competitive advantages.

HOW SHOULD AN HCO DEAL WITH THE MEDIA?

Media communication is either HCO initiated or media initiated. HCO-initiated communication is the planned release of information as part of branding or promotion of a specific service. Attractive, thorough releases; identification of visual elements for photos and television; access to knowledgeable, articulate spokespersons; and identification of newsworthy elements all assist in improving the coverage. A deliberate program of regular information releases and efforts to draw media attention to favorable events promote a positive image. The more information released, the greater the familiarity and attractiveness to the community.

Media-initiated communication is often related to events, such as treatment of prominent people or adverse occurrences either in or outside the HCO. Effective handling of media initiatives begins with preventing events that will draw investigation. It is supported by a strong branding program that releases newsworthy, positive information about the HCO. When unfortunate issues arise, the HCO should anticipate reporters' questions and prepare detailed, candid responses. Spokespersons should be identified and equipped with thorough, convincing replies to questions, within HIPAA confidentiality limits.

CAN PROMOTION CHANGE PATIENT BEHAVIOR?

Successful patient communication is a sophisticated combination of advertising, persuasion, and education. Three approaches improve its effectiveness:

1. Messages should be carefully targeted to specific population segments where change is desired—funds spent

communicating to populations that are uninvolved or non-responsive are wasted.

2. Advance plans for promotional campaigns should specify *reach* (the focal audience for the campaign), *frequency* (how often individuals in the focal audience are contacted), media, cost, and measures of expected outcome.

3. Campaigns should explicitly involve community partnerships and coalitions. Building networks improves solutions, reduces costs, builds mutual respect, and uses familiar faces to reach target audiences.

CAN PROMOTION CHANGE ASSOCIATE RECRUITMENT?

Most large HCOs promote themselves directly to clinical professionals in short supply. Programs to attract physicians are common. Many organizations advertise routinely in nursing, physical therapy, and pharmacy journals to attract new professionals.

Strategic affiliations to recruit personnel are also common. Affiliation with teaching programs enhances recruitment and retention of graduating students. Programs to assist students with summer and part-time work affect not only the students directly involved but also their classmates, who learn by word of mouth. Working with inner-city high schools to encourage young people to enter healing professions is popular. Like many promotional activities, it reaches two audiences—the students and the community at large. North Mississippi Medical Center operates a program beginning with "Let's Pretend Hospital, a tool to educate first graders in health care careers." Often current non-professional associates can advance to more skilled positions. Scholarships and scheduling assistance encourage such advancement.

ARE THE MISSION, VISION, AND VALUES DYNAMIC?

Even though major change is infrequent in the mission and even rarer in the vision and values, well-run organizations review the need for change annually. The organization should periodically undertake a broader-scale review, sometimes called "visioning." Actual revisions are developed by extensive listening and discussion among large numbers of stakeholders. Several task forces (often numbering in the hundreds of people) are established to attract representatives from most of the organization's stakeholders into debate about possible revisions. The review process strengthens consensus positions by focusing attention on the issues, increasing understanding of others' viewpoints, and clarifying the reasons for specific wording. Marketing must manage the task forces, keep track of proposed changes, and arrange for the resolution of serious disagreements. The final changes require formal governing board adoption.

HOW DOES THE HCO ESTABLISH ITS STRATEGIC POSITION?

As discussed in Chapter 1, the mission, vision, ownership, scope of services, location, and partners define the HCO's strategic position. Successful strategic positions are built around successful elements of current activity, by identifying and testing the alternatives with simulations and pilots and evaluating the tests in task forces or committees of the most knowledgeable stakeholders. It is almost impossible to start completely de novo; even new facilities with new visions must fit into competitive environments that shape them.

The governing board reviews the strategic position whenever necessary, but always as part of the annual environmental review. The fact-finding and analysis cover the dimensions of the strategic scorecard (exhibits 3.5 and 4.1), comparing achievements to expectations, competitors, and benchmarks. Comparison to excellent HCOs is helpful. Porter's framework for evaluating strategy is useful, both to improve the balanced scorecard measures and to identify important questions.[2] The framework suggests that strategy must address questions from "five forces" or external domains:

1. *Buyers and customers.* What are the needs of buyers, patients, and the community? What OFIs are revealed by benchmarking quality, cost, access, and amenities? What shortages or oversupply appear from the epidemiologic planning forecasts?

2. *New technology and substitutes.* What are the implications of new diagnostic and treatment technology? What opportunities exist to reduce the cost of technology, such as by substituting less expensive protocols or changing processes to use less skilled personnel? What opportunities for improvement are presented by new operational technology, such as the electronic medical record and guest guidance kiosks?

3. *Resource availability.* What funds are available for investment in expansion or renovation? What human resources are required, and how will they be acquired? What opportunities exist to improve retention and service excellence? What land is required? How effectively is the organization using its information resources?

4. *Competitor activity.* What actions are competitors taking, and what are the implications of those actions for our strategy? What opportunities exist to forward stakeholder goals by collaboration with competitors?

5. *Potential competitors and regulatory impact.* What new models of healthcare delivery are being developed elsewhere? Which stakeholder groups might start competing

---

[2]Porter, M. E. 1980. *Competitive Strategy: Techniques for Analyzing Industries and Competitors,* 4. New York: Free Press.

organizations, and why? What regulatory protections does the existing organization have? What incentives are offered to encourage competitors? What actions might our organization take to forestall competition?

The review helps a large number of associates understand the organization's profile of needs, achievements, and opportunities. The result is that the strategic position is not secret. In the words of the Intermountain Healthcare planner Greg Poulsen, "It's in our competitors' portfolio tomorrow morning."[3] The Intermountain approach is to win not on secrecy but on sound selection and effective implementation. Speed and thoroughness are both important.

The excellent HCOs used as models by *The Well-Managed Healthcare Organization* pursue comprehensive rather than niche strategies. They use transformational management, evidence-based management, and the service excellence model to build community-wide customer and provider brand loyalty. They counter niche competition with service lines and joint ventures offering niche services in integrated settings. They seek comprehensive coverage of market needs and are willing to explore multiple corporate and collaborative structures.

The HCO's strategic position is generally recorded in a group of interrelated documents:

- Environmental forecasts
- Services plan
- Facilities master plan
- Long-range financial plan
- Information services plan
- Human resources plan
- Medical staff plan

---

[3]Griffith, J. R., V. Sahney, and R. Mohr. 1995. *Reengineering Healthcare,* Chapter 4. Chicago: Health Administration Press.

Internal consulting is responsible for coordinating the strategic plans. The other technical and logistic support services are responsible for the plan components.

HOW DOES AN HCO DETERMINE ITS PARTNERSHIPS?

Leading HCOs recognize that "excellent care" must extend well beyond acute inpatient care, from primary care and telemedicine to continuing care and hospice. "Community health" as a mission (Chapter 9) requires an even broader focus. The model of transformational management and continuous improvement has been shown to be effective for all of these services. Underlying demand is forecast with the epidemiologic planning model. If the demand will support a viable entity, the question becomes, "How do we structure it?" Collaboration is often the best approach. "Collaborate" could mean "own," but it often includes other corporate structures. Exhibit 15.3 suggests several common levels of collaborative activity. The goal is to make high-quality, attractive, efficient services available to patients. Continuous improvement principles make that possible; the structure is a means to the end. Marketing and internal consulting analyze the pros and cons of alternative structures; senior management or governance does the negotiation; governance approves the final arrangement.

HOW ARE MARKETING AND STRATEGY ACTIVITIES IMPROVED?

Marketing and strategy processes are difficult to evaluate, but annual review, identification of OFIs, and deliberate improvement plans are still critical. The cost of current activities is easily tallied, and the contribution of most activities is evaluated by user

Exhibit 15.3 Spectrum of Potential Relationships with Organizations

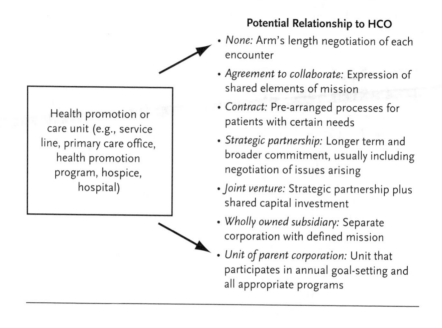

Health promotion or care unit (e.g., service line, primary care office, health promotion program, hospice, hospital)

Potential Relationship to HCO

- *None:* Arm's length negotiation of each encounter
- *Agreement to collaborate:* Expression of shared elements of mission
- *Contract:* Pre-arranged processes for patients with certain needs
- *Strategic partnership:* Longer term and broader commitment, usually including negotiation of issues arising
- *Joint venture:* Strategic partnership plus shared capital investment
- *Wholly owned subsidiary:* Separate corporation with defined mission
- *Unit of parent corporation:* Unit that participates in annual goal-setting and all appropriate programs

response, either survey, retention, or market share. However, the cost of an unexamined strategy—activities overlooked—can be catastrophic. User response does not reliably address activities that should have been undertaken but were not. Two avenues of review are especially critical:

1. Senior management and the governing board should take time after the environmental assessment and strategic goal-setting to reflect on the process, deliberately seeking consensus on penetrating questions:

    • How does our HCO compare to benchmark on cost, quality, and patient and associate satisfaction?

- Are there serious unmet customer needs or areas of dissatisfaction?
- Is there evidence of deterioration in customer support and satisfaction?
- Are direct competitors doing better than our HCO?
- Is there an unaddressed threat of human, financial, or physical resource shortage?
- Are there underutilized resources that could be converted to mission achievement?
- Did the HCO encounter unexpected events that it could have anticipated?

2. An audit performed by an outside consultant can review practices, goals, and organization structures and can suggest opportunities for improvement. Periodic use of an independent outsider will improve the reliability of internal review.

HOW MUCH SHOULD AN HCO SPEND ON MARKETING AND STRATEGY?

The amount of investment in strategy and marketing should be based on careful judgment. The question of how much to spend next year should conclude the review for improvements. Senior management and governance should be convinced that an adequate environmental assessment will be performed and that progress on major strategic agendas will be appropriate to long-term market needs. An HCO that cannot meet these conditions is a candidate for merger, acquisition, or closure.

CAN MULTI-HOSPITAL SYSTEMS CONTRIBUTE TO MARKETING AND STRATEGY?

The technical and leadership requirements for strategic excellence suggest a powerful advantage for large, multi-site healthcare systems.

The successful large healthcare system provides discipline and technical support in four critical areas:

1. Shaping mission, vision, and values to a comprehensive stakeholder perspective
2. Benchmarking the performance of all centralized processes; all logistic and strategic services should strive first to meet customer needs and second to minimize costs
3. Maintaining a listening and collaborative environment
4. Maintaining a learning environment

The models for the 21st century are with us today. Catholic Health Initiatives, SSM Health Care, and Intermountain Healthcare have exploited the possibilities and can document their superiority on the strategic scorecard. Others are joining them, but they are too little recognized, too seldom copied, and too often ignored.

SUGGESTED READINGS

Fortenberry, Jr., J. L. 2009. *Health Care Marketing: Tools and Techniques,* 3rd edition. Boston: Jones and Bartlett Publishers.

Kotler, P., J. Shalowitz, and R. J. Stevens. 2008. *Strategic Marketing for Health Care Organizations: Building a Customer-Driven Health System.* San Francisco: Jossey-Bass.

Porter, M. E. 2008. *On Competition.* Boston: Harvard Business School Publishing.

Swayne, L. E., J. Duncan, and P. M. Ginter. 2009. *Strategic Management of Health Care Organizations,* 6th edition. San Francisco: Jossey-Bass.

INDEX

Benchmarking/benchmarks, 22; of clinical support services, 151–152, 157, 159, 164; cost of, 37; for customer service, 37; as educational process, 119; for environment-of-care services, 261; hierarchical, 288; for knowledge management, 48–49, 201, 203; of operational infrastructure functions, 25, 26; performance below, 82; reliable, identification of, 288; standardized measures in, 49

Benefits management, 228, 232

Best practices, 48

Beverly Enterprises, 111

Board of Governors Examination in Healthcare Management, 9

Bonuses, 23, 24, 237–238

Boundary-spanning activities, 39, 54, 58

Branding, 313, 314, 318

Breast cancer screening programs, 95

Bronson Methodist Hospital, Kalamazoo, Michigan, 20, 251

Budget managers, 165

Budget process, 164–165. *See also* Financial management

Buffalo County Community Partners, community health program of, 189–192

Calendars: annual planning, 35, 40, 42, 43; of governing boards, 32, 63, 66

California, nurse staffing level regulations, 143

Cancer screening programs, 95

Capital investment proposals: preparation of, 293–294, 297; review of, 274–275, 294–296, 298

Capital investments, 164, 166; in community health, 195, 197; implementation of, 267

Cardiac surgery, physician organizations in, 117

Cardiovascular disease, care protocols for, 95

Career development, 235–236

Catholic Health Initiatives: community health investments of, 195, 197; strategic scorecard of, 326; trustee training program of, 70, 71

"Caught in the act" reports, 313–314, 316

Center for Health Care Strategies, 185

Centers for Disease Control and Prevention (CDC), 257; Task Force on Community Preventive Services, 177, 182, 192, 195

Centers for Medicare & Medicaid Services, MDS 3.0 program of, 186

Certification, continued, 111

Change: in healthcare, 107–108; process of, 15; in transition to excellence, 6

Chief executive officers (CEOs), performance evaluation of, 68

Chief financial officers (CFIs), 277–278

Chief information officers (CIOs), 201

Chief nursing officers (CNOs), 129

Child care protocols, 95

Chronic disease management, 177

Clinical information, 47

Clinical performance: improvement of, 85; monitoring of, 106

Clinical practice: guidelines for, 90–91; scale of, 120; systems-based, 110, 111, 119

Clinical protocol review teams, 89

Clinical protocols: advantages of, 86–87; definition of, 86; development of, 91, 119; functional, 86, 89–90, 92, 95, 159, 160, 166, 169–170; implementation of, 91–93; interdisciplinary plan of care as, 87–89; misunderstanding the applications of, 130; negotiation of, 30, 31; patient management, 87, 90–91, 92, 95, 159; physician organizations and, 106; pilot-tested, 83; reviewing of, 209; standards for, 81

Clinical services: operational scorecard template for, 96, 98–99; optimal size of, 50–51, 52; planning of, 82

Clinical support services. *See* Support services

Coaching, 18, 141

Coding, diagnostic, 210–211, 277

Collaboration: in community health, 187–188; with competitors, 187, 189; types of, 323, 324

Colleagues, performance evaluation of, 106

Collective bargaining, 228

College of American Pathologists, 166, 169

Commission to Build a Healthier America, 177

Commitment: consistent, 18, 22; to mission statement, 108

Communication, with media, 318

Communication skills, of physicians, 110, 119

Communications plan, in community health, 188–189

Communication systems, redundancy of, 248

Community, interactions with HCOs, 51, 53

Community care, as physician organization purpose, 108

Community health, 84, 85, 175–199; *versus* acute care, 195, 197; benefits of, 178–179; communications plan in, 188–189; community approach to, 186–189; conflict of interests related to, 178; continuous improvement of, 192–195; cost-effectiveness of, 182, 192, 193–194; definition of, 176; financial aspects of, 195, 197–198; frequently asked questions about, 197–198; as HCO mission, 93–95; implementation of, 179, 180–181; mature plans in, 189–192; needs assessment of, 179, 182–186; performance measures of, 192–195, 196, 308, 309; promotion of, 192

Community listening activities, 75

Community satisfaction, surveys of, 315

Community service, 17–18, 19, 20, 21, 39, 53

Compensation. *See also* Income: for clinical support service associates, 156, 157, 159; competitive, 163; incentive, 120, 237–238; negotiation of, 31; in service recovery, 236–237

Competency: credentialing-based, 100; maintenance of, 108; training-based, 86

Competition, 11; for clinical support services, 156, 157; niche, 322

Competitors: acquisition of, 308, 309; collaboration with, 187, 189; in community health, 187, 189; observation of, 317; strategic positioning implications of, 321

Complaints, 234, 313–314, 316

Compliance: corporate, 66; regulatory, 290

Complications, prevention of, 132, 135, 138

Confidentiality, 204, 206, 318

Conflict of interest: community health-related, 178; of consultants, 284; of governance board members, 62, 67

Conflict resolution, 42, 44, 101; as medical staff bylaw component, 122; with physician organizations, 125; physicians' participation in, 124

Consent agenda, 64

Consortia, 45–46, 299

Consultants. *See also* Internal consultants: for clinical performance improvement councils, 83; external, 286, 292, 299–300; for physician organization reviews, 125

Consultations, as clinical support service function, 158, 162

Continuing education, 24–25; of governing board members, 66; as physician organization function, 109; of physicians, 119

Continuous improvement, 18, 22; annual cycle of, 268; of clinical support services, 155, 158; of community health services, 192–195; effect on medical error rate, 100; of governing boards, 63; human resource management's role in, 228, 239, 240; infrastructure support for, 40–44; of knowledge management services, 205, 211, 214–216; as operational infrastructure function, 38; as operational infrastructure measure, 54, 56, 58; physician collaboration in, 109; training in, 291–292

Contractors, of knowledge management services, 218

Contracts: for clinical support services, 152, 154–159, 172; for community health services, 188; for construction and renovation, 251, 252; for consulting, 286; for environment-of-care services, 252–253; physician–HCO, 119–120; for workers' compensation insurance, 233

Control charts, 289–290
Coordination, as operational infrastructure, 38, 42
Core values, 93
Corporate design, 45–47
Cost accounting, 261–262
Cost analysis, 273
Cost improvement, 35
Credentialing, 106, 108; of clinical support service associates, 155; as competency guarantee, 86, 113; process of, 113–115; programs in, 81, 100
Crime prevention, 249
Cultural competence, 230, 231–232
Cultural foundation, of excellence, 7, 8, 92
Culture, empowerment/transformational, 13–33; backlash against, 23; definition of, 14–15; effectiveness of, 16–17; establishment of, 17–23; expansion of, 23–24; improvement of, 24; measurement of, 24–27; nurses' implementation of, 141; sustaining of, 23–24
Customer satisfaction. See also Patient satisfaction: with accounting services, 280

Dashboards, 42. See also Scorecards: for governing board evaluation, 65, 66
Data warehouses, 38, 208, 209
DaVita, 111
Deadlines, 42
Decision making: operational, 284; physicians' participation in, 122, 123; strategic, 284
Decision support, 47, 48
Deming, W. Edwards, 208
Demonstration sites, 18
Design, of healthcare facilities, 251
Diabetes, care protocols for, 95
Diagnoses: accurate, 81, 84, 85, 86; support services for, 81
Diagnosis-related groups (DRGs), 210, 217, 276–277
Disaster/emergency preparedness and response, 53, 249, 257–259
Discharge, of patients, 137, 139

Disease prevention programs, 84, 93–95, 177, 178, 189; cost-effectiveness of, 182; levels of, 182
Dismissal, of incompetent employees, 235
Disputes, negotiation of, 29–32. See also Conflict resolution
Diversity: in leadership, 25; promotion of, 225; in the workplace, 225, 230, 231–232
Due diligence, 77

Educational programs, for governing board members, 61, 71–72
Electronic health records (EHRs), 47, 50; implementation of, 101
Emergency preparedness and response. See Disaster/emergency preparedness and response
Employee information centers, 48
Employees, behavior standards for, 27–29, 277–278
Employers, involvement in community health, 187
Empowerment, 13, 15, 16, 224; of external stakeholders, 75–76; of internal stakeholders, 75; of physicians, 122
Environmental assessment, 267, 268, 270, 287–288, 320
Environmental Protection Agency (EPA), 248
Environmental review. See Environmental assessment
Environment-of-care management (ECM), 245–263; comparison with Ritz-Carlton, 245, 248–249; components of, 247; construction and renovation component of, 251–252, 299; contractors for, 247; cost control in, 261–262; cost of, 246, 248, 254, 255–256; design component of, 251; goals of, 247–248; hazardous materials control component of, 233, 248, 254; improvement of, 259–261; materials management functions of, 254–256; purposes of, 247; risk management and, 246, 256–257; service provision for, 252–254; space allocation component of, 249–251

Epidemiologic planning model, 50–51, 52, 96, 99; for clinical support service demand, 157; internal consultants' responsibility for, 288; for physician organizations, 116; for space allocation, 249

Equity, 29, 32

Errors. *See also* Unexpected events: knowledge-based reduction of, 217; response to, 100–101

Ethical conflicts, in community health, 198

Ethics committees, 88–89, 92, 290

Evidence-based approach, to excellence, 4

Evidence-based culture, 69

Evidence-based management, 22, 284–285

Evidence-based medicine, 83, 107, 111

Evidence-based nursing, 137–138

Excellence: achievement of, 84; definition of, 4–5; obstacles to, 2–3, 100–102

Excellent healthcare organizations, 2. *See also* Healthcare organizations (HCOs): characteristics of, 5–6, 83–84; foundations of, 7, 8; number of, 5

Exceptional effort, reports of, 313–314, 316

Excise taxes, 67

Exit interviews, 236

Faith-based organizations, 187

Faith-based restrictions, on healthcare, 198

Federally qualified health centers (FQHCs), 185

Fee-for-service payment, 119

Fellows, of American College of Healthcare Executives, 9

Finance personnel, 277–278

Finance system, purposes of, 267

Financial information, 48

Financial management, 83, 266–281; auditing in, 276, 277; "backstage" activities in, 267; capital investment evaluation in, 274–275; cost analysis in, 273; forecasting in, 273; goal-setting in, 269–272; indirect cost management in, 266; "onstage" activities in, 267–268, 278–279; operating unit performance reports in, 272; overhead cost control in, 275–276

Financial planning, long-range, 74, 268–269, 288

Financial support, 16

Focus groups, 188, 317

Food services, 249

Forecasting, 273, 287, 288, 289

Foster McGaw Prize, 177

Functional protocols, 86, 89–90, 92, 159, 160, 166, 169–170

Gain-sharing, 223, 237–238

Goal(s): of excellent healthcare organizations, 5; financial, 268–269; negotiation of, 267; operational, 269–272; quantitative, 44; strategic, 269–272; "stretch," 237

Goal achievement: incentive compensation for, 237–238; ninety-day plans for, 38; timetables for, 38, 76–77

Goal setting, 22; annual, 38, 39; by clinical support services, 164–166; coordination and integration in, 42; financial, 268–272; for future goals, 76; by governing board, 40; information use in, 209; operational, 269–272; process of, 77; strategic, 267, 269–272

Governance. *See also* Governing board: in distressed conditions, 77–78; excellent, definition of, 63–64

Governing board, 17, 18, 61–79; calendar of, 32, 63, 66; corporate governance committee of, 67; effectiveness measures of, 64–69; functions of, 63–64; goal-setting function of, 268–269; internal members of, 75; knowledge management review role of, 214, 216; members' conflicts of interest, 62, 67; membership, 62, 122, 124–125; performance improvement of, 72–78; physician members of, 122, 124–125; recruitment of members, 70; self-evaluation of, 67

Grievance management, 234

Harassment, 146

Hazardous materials management, 233, 248, 254

HCOs. *See* Healthcare organizations (HCOs)

Joint ventures, 39, 45, 46–47; in community health, 189; as niche competition response, 322; physician–HCO, 120

Justice, as community health issue, 198

Just-in-time services, 256

Just-in-time support, 286

Just-in-time training, 49, 209–210, 292

Kansas University Work Group for Community Health and Development, 177

Key performance indicators, 48

Knowledge management, 54, 57, 69, 201–219; "backstage" duties in, 202, 203, 204–206, 208, 218; benchmarking in, 48–49; continuous improvement of, 205, 211, 214–216; financing of, 202–203, 216, 217; "onstage" duties in, 203, 204, 209–211, 218; as operational infrastructure component, 38; performance measures of, 211, 212–213; planning committees in, 214, 215–216, 218; problems in, 202–204; purpose of, 203; vendors and contractors in, 218

Knowledge management network, 47–50

Knowledge resource, 203–204

Layoffs, 233–234

Leadership education, 119

Leaders/leadership: accountability of, 25; development and training of, 235–236, 292–293; diversity in, 25; of expansion sites, 23; physicians as, 114; responsive, 17, 18, 27–29, 32–33; of transformational culture, 23

Lean manufacturing, 42, 119, 292–293

Leapfrog Group, 97

Learning, practice-based, 110–111

Linguistic services, 232

Listening: in collaborative activities, 187; as marketing component, 31, 313–314, 315–317; to patients, 88; responsive, 131, 170, 224; to stakeholders, 31, 313–314, 315–317; systematic, 53, 54

Listening skills, 29

Loyalty: of customers, 236; job security and, 230; of medical staff, 120–125

Magnet Recognition Program, 129–130, 132

Malcolm Baldrige National Quality Award recipients, 5, 11; mission statements, vision statements, and values of, 19–21; physician organizations of, 106–107; Ritz-Carlton, 245, 248–249

Malpractice, 23, 83, 101, 132, 237

Management excellence, elements of, 9–10

Managers: community service involvement, 53; finance/accounting, 277–278; human resource management support for, 224–225; interaction with clinical support services, 170–172; on-call, 317

Marketing, 111, 307–327; of community health programs, 192; definition of, 309, 310; external review of, 325; "four Ps" of, 310, 313; functions of, 311–312; improvement of, 323–325; internal review of, 323–325; investments in, 325; by multi-hospital systems, 326; purpose of, 309; segmentation in, 207, 313; social, 192; technical requirements for, 309–310

Market share, 102, 307, 308

Materials management functions, 254–256

Media, interactions with, 318

Medical Executive Committee, 11

Medical knowledge, of physicians, 110–111

Medicare, 6

Medication administration protocols, 90

Mediocrity, 73–74

Mentoring, 24–25, 141, 236

Mercy Health System: annual planning calendar of, 43; mission statements, vision statements, and values of, 21

Mergers, 308

Mission statements, 17; of Baldrige Award recipients, 19–21; contributions to, 22, 123; review and revision of, 320

Modeling, 18

Mortality rates, adjustment of, 207

Mystery shopping, 317

Patient care, physicians' competency in, 110–111

Patient-centered care, 85

Patient records, automated, 38. *See also* Electronic health records

Patient satisfaction, 15, 16, 23; with clinical support services, 151, 168, 169–170; with nursing care, 131, 148; surveys of, 24, 122, 315

Patient scheduling: for clinical support services, 159, 160–162; nurses' role in, 143, 144

Performance evaluations: as educational process, 119; of governing boards, 64, 65

Performance improvement councils (PICs), 11, 35, 53; clinical protocol improvement role of, 92; for clinical support services, 160; for financial goal-setting, 271; internal consultants' assistance to, 292; in knowledge management, 201; supervisory function of, 40

Performance improvement teams (PITs): clinical, effectiveness of, 82–83; clinical performance improvement role of, 96; in clinical support services, 151, 152, 170, 171; control of decision making, 300–301; of environment-of-care services, 253, 254; in financial goal-setting, 271, 273; functional protocol review role of, 89, 91; internal consultants' assistance to, 292; knowledge support for, 201; membership of, 82, 83; supervision of, 40; technical assistance to, 42; timetables for, 42, 82

Performance measures, 47–50, 96–97, 98; adjustment of, 207, 208, 289; clinical, 96–97, 99; of clinical support services, 166–169; of community health programs, 192–195, 196; financial, 272; for human resources management, 239, 242; of nursing care, 145, 147–148; of operational infrastructure functions, 56–58; random variability of, 207, 208; random variation of, 201, 207, 208; reliability of, 202, 206; standardization of, 289; statistical process control of, 289–290

Performance reviews, 360-degree (multi-rater), 24–25

PERT (program evaluation and review technique), 298

Physician-healthcare organization relationship, frequently asked questions about, 106–107

Physician information center, 47

Physician organizations (POs), 105–127; functions of, 108, 109; improvement of, 125–126; of Malcolm Baldrige Award recipients, 105–127; physician incomes in, 119–120; physician supply for, 115–118; role in excellent healthcare, 111–113

Physicians: competencies of, 110–111; oversupply of, 115, 116, 118; relationship with HCOs, 81; shortage of, 115, 116, 118; as team leaders, 107

Physician satisfaction, 108, 122; with clinical support services, 168; monitoring of, 125, 126; with nursing care, 148

PICs. *See* Performance improvement councils (PICs)

Picture archive and communication systems (PACs), 47

Pilots, in cultural transformation, 18, 22

Pilot testing: of clinical protocols, 83; of proposed process revisions, 292

PITs. *See* Performance improvement teams (PITs)

Planning, 54; of clinical services, 82; as governing board's function, 68

Postnatal care protocols, 95

Poudre Valley Health System (PVHS): knowledge management network of, 47–50; mission statements, vision statements, and values of, 21

Poulsen, Greg, 322

Power, knowledge-based, 27

Prenatal care protocols, 95

Preventive healthcare programs, 53, 93–95

Price, as marketing component, 313

Primary care, as specialist income support, 105–106

Primary care physicians, shortage of, 116

Primary prevention, 94, 95, 182, 183

Sensitivity analysis, 289
Servant leaders, 17
Service excellence, 15, 16, 23, 224; goal of, 17; as leadership context, 25–27
Service lines: accountability for revenue, 276–277; clinical, 96, 97; functional protocols and, 92; functions of, 85; patient management protocols and, 90; support services for, 111–113
Service recovery, 236–237, 313–314, 316
Sexual harassment, 232–233
Shadowing, 317
Sharp HealthCare, San Diego, 5; community interactions of, 51, 53; employee behavior standards of, 277–278; knowledge management criteria of, 206; mission statements, vision statements, and values of, 21; positive reinforcement use by, 27
Significance level, 208
Six Sigma, 42, 119, 292–293
Smoking bans, 189
Software: for information capture, 206; management of, 204; for statistical process control, 208
Space allocation, 249–251
Specialists, 102
Specification, 206, 207, 289
SSM Health Care: community health investments of, 195, 197; mission statements, vision statements, and values of, 19; strategic scorecard of, 326
Staffing: nursing, 23, 30, 131, 132, 137, 142–145, 146, 222; operational infrastructure and, 39; planning for, 39
Stakeholders: equal treatment of, 29, 32; HCO interactions with, 51, 53; monitoring of needs of, 39; satisfaction of, 58
Standard deviation, 208
Standard error, 208
Standards of care, 170
Statistical process control, 201, 207–208, 289–290, 316
Strategic activities: external review of, 325; internal review of, 323–325; of multi-hospital systems, 326
Strategic cost, 268–269

Strategic foundation, of excellence, 7, 8, 39
Strategic positioning, 76, 111, 288; documentation of, 322; establishment of, 320–323; external domains of, 321–322; review/evaluation of, 320–322
Strategic support services, 102
Strategy, 307–327; definition of, 309–310; functions of, 312; investments in, 325; processes of, 323–325; technical requirements for, 309–310
Subcommittees, 62, 72, 75
Subpopulations, 207
Subsidiaries, 39, 46–47
Substance abuse recovery programs, 114–115
Succession plans, 230
Supply chain, 254–256
Support services, 38, 151–173; affiliations with HCOs, 169; contracts with HCOs, 154–159; core organization of, 171; customers of, 162–163; for diagnosis, 81; of excellent HCOs, 106–107; functional protocols of, 166, 169–170; functions of, 159–160; of integrated HCOs, 111; integration into interdisciplinary plans of care, 159; negotiation with, 164–166; for nurses, 145, 146; nurses' role in, 140; ownership of, 169; performance measures of, 151, 166–169, 167–168; purpose of, 153; service line requirements for, 111–113; size of, 51; vendor-provided, 111
Surveys, of patient, associate, and community satisfaction, 315
Sustaining, of operational infrastructure, 58
Systems analysis, 42
Systems-based clinical practice, 110, 111, 119

Task Force on Community Preventive Services, 177, 182, 192, 195
Team approach, in healthcare, 107, 111
Team units, 22
Telemedicine, 102
Temporary employees, 229
Tertiary prevention, 95, 182, 183
Theft, 256

ABOUT THE AUTHORS

John R. Griffith, MBA, FACHE, is the Andrew Pattullo Collegiate Professor in the Department of Health Management and Policy at the School of Public Health, the University of Michigan, Ann Arbor. A graduate of The Johns Hopkins University and the University of Chicago, he was director of the Program and Bureau of Hospital Administration at the University of Michigan from 1970 to 1982 and was the chair of his department from 1987 to 1991.

Professor Griffith has served as chair of the Association of University Programs in Health Administration (AUPHA), as a commissioner for the Accrediting Commission on Education in Health Services Administration, and as senior advisor to the board of the National Center for Healthcare Leadership.

The seventh edition of *The Well-Managed Healthcare Organization*, which Professor Griffith authored with Kenneth R. White, PhD, FACHE, has been called the "definitive resource" on the subject. The first edition won the American College of Healthcare Executives Hamilton Award for book of the year in 1987. The fourth edition was recognized by the Healthcare Information and Management Systems Society as the 2000 book of the year. Professor Griffith also authored two articles in the *Journal of Health Administration Education* on the implications of competency assessment in graduate education, titled "Improving Preparation for Senior Management in Health Care" and "Advancing Education for Evidence-Based Healthcare Management."

Professor Griffith was awarded ACHE's Gold Medal Award in 1992. He was also recognized with the John Mannix Award of the Cleveland Hospital Council, the Edgar Hayhow Award (in 1989, 2003, and 2006) and Dean Conley Prizes of ACHE, AUPHA's Filerman Prize for Educational Excellence, and citations from the Michigan Hospital Association and the Governor of Michigan. He received the Excellence in Teaching Award from the University of Michigan School of Public Health in 2009. He was an examiner for the Malcolm Baldrige National Quality Award from 1997 to 1998.

Kenneth R. White, PhD, FACHE, has more than 35 years of experience in healthcare organizations in clinical, administrative, governance, academic, and consulting capacities. He spent 13 years with Mercy Health Services as a senior executive in marketing, operations, and international healthcare consulting.

From 1995 to 2001, Dr. White served as the associate director of the graduate programs in health administration (MHA and MSHA) at Virginia Commonwealth University (VCU). From 2001 to 2008, he served as the director of VCU's Master of Health Administration and Dual Degree (MHA/JD and MHA/MD) programs. From 2006 to 2009, he served as VCU's first Charles P. Cardwell, Jr. Professor. At VCU, he holds a joint appointment as professor of nursing and visiting professor of the Luiss Guido Carli University in Rome, Italy, and the Swiss School of Public Health in Lugano, Switzerland.

Dr. White is a registered nurse and a Fellow and former member of the Board of Governors of the American College of Healthcare Executives. He has served on several hospital and health system boards as well.

Dr. White received a PhD in health services organization and research from VCU. He earned an MPH in health administration from the University of Oklahoma and an MS in nursing from VCU. He has extensive experience in hospital administration and consulting, particularly in the areas of leadership development, marketing, facility planning, and management of operations.

He is coauthor (with John R. Griffith) of *The Well-Managed Healthcare Organization*, 5th, 6th, and 7th editions; *Thinking Forward: Six Strategies for Successful Organizations; and Reaching Excellence in Healthcare Management* (all published by Health Administration Press). Dr. White is a contributing author to the book *Human Resources in Healthcare: Managing for Success and Evidence-Based Management in Healthcare* (Health Administration Press). He is also a contributing author to the books *Advances in Health Care Organization Theory* (Jossey-Bass), *Peri-Anesthesia Nursing: A Critical Care Approach* (Saunders), *On the Edge: Nursing in the Edge of Complexity,* and *Introduction to Health Services* (Delmar).

Dr. White was given ACHE's Edgar C. Hayhow Award in 2006 for his article (with John Griffith) "The Revolution in Hospital Management," published in the *Journal of Healthcare Management*. Dr. White has received ACHE's Distinguished Service Award and two Regent's Awards (1999 and 2010) and the Virginia Nurses Association's "Virginia's Outstanding Nurse" award (1999). At VCU, Dr. White has earned the President's Award for Multicultural Enrichment and numerous teaching awards.